Hormonal Proteins and Peptides

VOLUME V
Lipotropin and Related Peptides

Contributors

M. Chrétien
C. W. Jones
Choh Hao Li
M. Lis
B. T. Pickering
Jerker Porath

HORMONAL PROTEINS AND PEPTIDES

Edited by CHOH HAO LI

The Hormone Research Laboratory
University of California
San Francisco, California

VOLUME V
Lipotropin and Related Peptides

ACADEMIC PRESS New York San Francisco London 1978
A Subsidiary of Harcourt Brace Jovanovich, Publishers

ACADEMIC PRESS, INC.
111 Fifth Avenue, New York, New York 10003

United Kingdom Edition published by
ACADEMIC PRESS, INC. (LONDON) LTD.
24/28 Oval Road, London NW1

Library of Congress Cataloging in Publication Data

Li, Choh Hao, Date
Hormonal proteins and peptides.

Vol. 5 has also special title: Lipotropin and related peptides.
Includes bibliographies.
1. Protein hormones—Collected works. 2. Peptide hormones—Collected works. I. Title. [DNLM: 1. Hormones. 2. Peptides. 3. Proteins. QU55 L693h]
QP572.P77L5 599'.01'927 72-88367
ISBN 0-12-447205-2(v.5)

PRINTED IN THE UNITED STATES OF AMERICA

Contents

List of Contributors

Numbers in parentheses indicate the pages on which the authors' contributions begin.

M. Chrétien (75), Protein and Polypeptide Hormone Laboratory, Clinical Research Institute of Montreal, Montreal, Quebec, Canada

C. W. Jones* (103), Department of Physiology and Pharmacology, University of Nottingham, Nottingham, England

Choh Hao Li (1, 35), Hormone Research Laboratory, University of California, San Francisco, California

M. Lis (75), Laboratory of Comparative Endocrinology, Clinical Research Institute of Montreal, Montreal, Quebec, Canada

B. T. Pickering (103), Department of Anatomy, University of Bristol, Bristol, England

Jerker Porath (159), Institute of Biochemistry, University of Uppsala, Uppsala, Sweden

* Present address: Medical Department, Syntex Pharmaceuticals Ltd., Maidenhead, England.

Preface

The first four chapters of this volume deal with peptides having neurobiological properties. For a long time, melanotropins have been known to control color changes chiefly in lower vertebrates. It has now been discovered that melanotropins, corticotropin, and their peptide fragments affect the behavior of rats and human subjects. The first chapter reviews the present knowledge of the chemistry of melanotropins.

Late in December 1975, metenkephalin was isolated in mammalian brain extracts and was shown to exhibit morphinelike activity. This led to the discovery of endorphins from pituitary glands. The second chapter presents the current knowledge of the most potent morphinelike peptide, β-endorphin. It is of interest to note that β-melanotropin, metenkephalin, and β-endorphin have amino acid sequences in the primary structure of β-lipotropin. In the third chapter, Chrétien and Lis summarize the chemistry and biology of lipotropins which were discovered and characterized in 1964–1965. It took more than ten years to realize the biologic significance of this pituitary hormone.

In the fourth chapter, Pickering and Jones review extensively and critically the properties and physiological role of neurophysins. Like β-lipotropin, neurophysin was discovered by Van Dyke and his colleagues in 1942, and its importance as a carrier for posterior pituitary hormones was recognized thirteen years later.

The prerequisite for the study of the structure and function of any natural product is its isolation in pure form. It is therefore important to devise effective methods for this purpose. Tiselius and his pupils have focused on the separation techniques for proteins and peptides for many years. Their contributions play an essential role in the development of protein chemistry. In the final chapter, Porath presents a historical perspective of the achievements of the Uppsala School, with a biographical sketch of Tiselius. Porath was one of Tiselius's favorite pupils, and is a coinventor of Sephadex, which has been widely used in chemical and biochemical laboratories.

I am indebted to the authors and to the staff of Academic Press for their cooperation in the preparation of this volume.

Choh Hao Li

Contents of Previous Volumes

1

The Chemistry of Melanotropins

CHOH HAO LI

I. Introduction

In 1916, Smith and Allen independently reported a striking change in the pigmentation of the tadpole following hypophysectomy. According to Smith (1916, 1919), the removal of the hypophysis in the tadpole is followed by a decrease in the amount of intracellular melanin, as well as in the number of the epidermal melanophores. Subsequently, Allen (1920) and Swingle (1921) showed that transplantation of the intermediate lobe of adult frogs into normal or hypophysectomized tadpoles causes a marked expansion of the melanocytes. Smith and Smith (1923) further demonstrated that extracts of the intermediate lobes of the bovine pituitary exercised the most marked influence on the pigmentation of the hypophysectomized tadpole, although suspensions of the anterior lobes were also effective in this regard. These earlier investigations leave no doubt that the pituitary gland possesses a principle or principles which regulate the pigmentation of amphibia.

A. Terminology

In 1932, Zondek and Krohn studied the effect of bovine pituitary extracts on the appearance of erythrophores and concluded that a principle elaborated in the intermediate lobe was responsible for an increased formation of red pigment in the skin of *Phoxinus*. They proposed the name "intermedin" for the principle. Various other names have been coined for the hormone, including melanophore hormone, melanophore-dilating or -expanding hormones, chromatophorotropic hormone, melanophore-stimulating hormone, the B hormone, the melanosome-dispersing hormone, and the pigmentation hormone. The term "melanocyte-stimulating hormone," or "MSH," was adopted by Lerner *et al*. (1954) after a suggestion by W. H. Rattner.

In 1957, Li proposed the term "melanotropin." This term has now been accepted by the Commission on Biochemical Nomenclature of the International Union of Pure and Applied Chemistry and the International Union of Biochemistry.*

B. Occurrence

Nearly all the experiments that have been carried out with amphibia have led to the conclusion that the intermediate lobe of the hypophysis is the site of origin of melanotropin. In the case of animals like the whale and the chicken in which the intermediate lobe of the pituitary is missing, melanocyte-stimulating activity can be extracted from the anterior lobe of the gland (Geiling, 1935, 1942). It has also been reported that the anterior lobe of the human pituitary is richer in melanotropin than is the intermediate lobe (area of basophil invasion) or the posterior lobe (Roth, 1932; Jores and Glogner, 1933). Steelman *et al*. (1956) have reported the presence of MSH in transplantable adrenotropic tumors in a concentration

* See *J. Biol. Chem.* **250**, 3215–3246 (1975).

equivalent to that in the normal mouse pituitary. It has been shown that tumors associated with "ectopic ACTH syndrome" contain at least two melanotropic substances (Steelman *et al.*, 1956).

C. Methods of Bioassay

The earlier methods for the biologic assay of melanotropin have been summarized by Landgrebe and Waring (1950). Most of the proposed methods may be classified into two groups: (a) the *in vivo* procedures, performed in either the intact or hypophysectomized frog, in which the dispersion of melanin granules in the melanophores of the web is observed microscopically and quantitated according to the melanophore index of Hogben and Slome (1931); and (b) the *in vitro* methods, whereby isolated segments of frog skin are placed in a solution of the hormone, and the degree of darkening is registered by a suitable photoelectric device. The specificity and sensitivity of these two procedures have been investigated in great detail by Thing (1952, 1953a,b).

For the routine assay of MSH activity, the *in vitro* method is convenient and simple to perform. Trendelenburg (1924) was probably the first to assay MSH activity by immersing isolated frog skin in a solution of the material to be tested. Wright (1946) and Frieden *et al*. (1948) have described quantitative techniques for determining the degree of darkening of the isolated frog skin in a measure of the melanotropic potency. The method of Shizume *et al*. (1954) can be said to have brought the *in vitro* assay procedure to a truly quantitative basis, making it amenable to statistical analysis (Lerner and Wright, 1960). This method depends upon the changes in light reflection (measured by a photoelectric reflection meter) from the skin of *Rana pipiens* frogs, produced by immersion of the skin in solutions containing MSH. Within certain limits (0.2–2.0 units), the logarithm of the hormonal concentration is proportional to the ratio of the changes in reflectance obtained with the unknown preparations and with 1 U/ml of the reference preparation. Recently, Ramachandran (1970) used a four-point design with quadruplicate observations and calculated the potency by variance analysis (Barth, 1960) using pure α_s-ACTH as the standard.

As yet, there is no established international standard unit of melanotropic potency. Shizume *et al*. (1954) tentatively defined as 1 unit the effect produced by 0.04 μg of a preparation obtained in their laboratory. Landgrebe and Waring (1950) have suggested that the same international reference standard that is officially accepted for pressor, oxytocic, and antidiuretic activity also be adopted for melanophore-expanding activity; i.e., that an international unit of MSH be defined as the amount of activity (determined by *in vivo* assay) present in 0.5 mg of the international standard posterior lobe power.

There are no published data for comparing the unit proposed by Shizume, Lerner, and Fitzpatrick (SLF) (1954) with that proposed by Landgrebe and Waring (LW) (1950). However, it has been determined that 1 LW unit is equivalent of 10^4 SLF units. In this chapter, the SLF unit will be used in reporting the activity of melanotropin.

The skins of lizards *(Anolis)* have been used for bioassay of melanotropins *in vivo* (Kleinholz and Rahn, 1940) and *in vitro* (Burgers, 1961; Bjorklund *et al.,* 1972). Tilders *et al.* (1975) reported in detail a simple and rapid assay procedure for the quantitative determination of melanotropic activity using skin fragments *in vitro* of the lizard *Anolis carolinensis* as previously described by Burgers (1961).

Radioimmunoassay techniques have been developed to measure minute quantities of melanotropins. Experimental generation of antibodies to α-MSH was first reported by McGuire *et al.* (1965) and Abe *et al.* (1967a). Recently, a sensitive and specific method for the measurement of immunoreactive α-MSH was reported by Usategni *et al.* (1976). The detection limit of their procedure was 6 pg/ml of plasma. These authors estimated the α-MSH content in the rat neurointermediate lobe to be 1930 ± 360 (SE) ng (Usategni *et al.,* 1976).

A radioimmunoassay method for β-MSH has also been developed for identification and quantification of this hormone in human plasma and tissues (Abe *et al.,* 1967b; Donnadien and Sevauz, 1974). By this method, Abe *et al.* (1967b) reported β-MSH concentrations in the plasma of normal subjects were less than 0.09 ng/ml.

D. Function of MSH in the Mammal

The precise function of melanotropin, except in amphibia and some fish, is not at all clear. It is thought by some to be concerned in visual adaptation (Jores, 1933). It has been claimed (Hanaoka, 1951) that MSH concentrates prepared from bovine, equine, and porcine pituitaries, when administered subcutaneously to human subjects, are active in shortening the time of adaptation to darkness and increasing sensitivity to light. It was further reported by the same author (Hanaoka, 1953) that the hormone is capable of accelerating regeneration of visual purple in the retina.

Mussio Fournier *et al.* (1936, 1943) have reported that, with MSH concentrates, repigmentation was effected in patients with vitiligo. Lerner *et al.* (1954), working with more highly purified MSH preparations, did not succeed in confirming this observation, although they demonstrated darkening of human skin and nevi and the formation of new nevi as a consequence of the administration of this hormone. The latter investigators also noted increased pigmentation within a few hours after the administration of large doses of hormone (Lerner and Takahashi, 1956).

Melanotropins have been shown to exert action on the central nervous system. Ferrari *et al.* (1963; Ferrari, 1958) reported that α-MSH causes stretching and yawning movements in dogs. β-Melanotropin enhances the amplitude of spinal cord monosynaptic potentials (Krivoy and Guillemin, 1961). Long *et al.* (1961) postulated that melanotropins play a role in central neural control. In rats, α-MSH exhibits an inhibitory effect on extinction of conditioned avoidance behavior (De Wied, 1966; De Wied and Bohns, 1966). Sandman *et al.* (1971, 1972) also reported that melanotropins have effects on attention, memory, and certain aspects of learning behavior. Two observed effects of β-MSH on rodents resemble the effects of catecholamines. These are behavioral changes, namely, hyperexcitability in mice and lethargy in rats (Sakamoto, 1966), and radioprotection to lethal whole body x-irradiation (Sakamoto and Prasad, 1967).

The effects of α- and β-MSH on the thyroid were studied in mice injected with ^{131}I and pretreated with thyroxine by Bowers *et al.* (1964). It was found that melanotropins cause an increase in blood levels of ^{131}I, as well as the uptake of ^{131}I. Melanotropins were found also to stimulate thyroid activity in rabbits (Courrier and Cehovic, 1960) and in guinea pigs (Cehovic, 1962).

α-MSH was shown to act synergistically with testosterone and to stimulate the sebaceous, prostate, and preputial glands and the seminal vesicles in hypophysectomized–castrated rats (Ebling *et al.*, 1975; Thody and Shuster, 1975; Thody *et al.*, 1976). Ebling *et al.* (1975) also showed that α-MSH not only acted synergistically, but also had a significant effect on the sebaceous glands, and this effect was independent of the presence of exogenous testosterone. Thody and Shuster (1975) found that α-MSH acts synergistically with progesterone to stimulate sebum secretion. These authors suggest that α-MSH acts directly on the sebaceous glands to stimulate lipogenesis, and, together with steroid hormones, may have an important role in controlling sebaceous gland function in the rat and other hairy mammals. Thody and Shuster (1973, 1975) further propose that, with the evolution of hair, certain of the melanotropin peptides may have lost their significance as pigmentary hormones and have developed a sebotropic function and that melanotropins may be referred to as "sebotropins."

Injections of relatively large doses of α- and β-MSH can cause skin darkening in man (Lerner and McGuire, 1961; McGuire and Lerner, 1963). The epidermal melanocytes of guinea pigs (Snell, 1962), weasel (Rust, 1965), and mouse (Geschwind *et al.*, 1972) are effected by administration of melanotropins. Geschwind and Huseby (1966) reported that a darkening coat color occurred in mice bearing an MSH-secreting pituitary tumor. For mechanism of action and regulation of melanotropin release, readers may refer to two recent reviewers (Howe, 1973; Hadley and Bagnara, 1975).

II. Preparation of Melanotropin Concentrate and Isolation of Porcine β-MSH

The posterior lobes of beef and pig pituitary glands have been the main source of starting material for the purification of melanotropins. Earlier research on methods for the preparation of extracts rich in MSH activity has been reviewed by Van Dyke (1936) and Landgrebe *et al.* (1955). In the early 1950's, a renewed interest in the isolation of melanotropins, stemming from the speculation that corticotropin and melanotropin may be identical, has stimulated intensive efforts that led to the isolation of porcine and bovine melanotropins in pure form. During this period, all the published procedures for the preparation of MSH concentrates from either porcine or bovine posterior pituitaries incorporate the acetic acid extraction technique first introduced by Kamm *et al.* (1928) for posterior pituitary hormones. The following, employed routinely in this laboratory for the preparation of porcine, bovine, or ovine MSH concentrates (Geschwind and Li, 1957) is an example of such a procedure.

Acetone-dried porcine posterior pituitary powder (200 gm), with an average activity of 2×10^4 unit/mg, was wetted with 500 ml of acetone and then extracted with 2 liters of glacial acetic acid at 50° for 20 minutes. The mixture was centrifuged, and the precipitate was reextracted with 400 ml of acetic acid, followed by 400 ml of acetone. To the combined extracts, 20 ml of saturated aqueous NaCl was added, followed by half a volume of acetone. The solution was stirred and then allowed to stand for 1 hour in an ice bath. After centrifugation, 1 volume of diethyl ether was added to the clear supernatant fluid; the ether solution was stirred and returned to the ice bath for 2 hours. The clear supernatant fluid was siphoned off, and the precipitate was washed extensively with acetone. The washed precipitate was transferred to a desiccator over NaOH. The average yield was 44 gm of material with an average activity of 5×10^4 units/mg.

The dried ether precipitate was dissolved with stirring in 1500 ml of 0.1 *N* acetic acid; to the clear solution (any insoluble material being removed by centrifugation), 6 gm of oxycellulose (10–12% COOH) was added, and the resulting suspension was stirred overnight. The suspension was then centrifuged, and the oxycellulose obtained in this manner was washed twice with 0.1 *N* acetic acid and once with water. The adsorbed MSH activity was eluted from the washed oxycellulose with 150 ml of 0.1 *N* HCl for 1 hour. When the eluate was submitted to centrifugation, a clear extract was obtained. The precipitate was reextracted for 30 minutes with 100 ml of 0.1 *N* HCl, and the two extracts were combined. These combined extracts were deacidified and lyophilized. The lyophilized powder (average yield, 600 mg) was then dissolved in 30 ml of water, and the pH of the solution was adjusted to 6.5–7.0 with NH_4OH. The resulting precipitate was removed by centrifugation, and the supernatant fluid was lyophilized. The average yield of this crude MSH concentrate from 200 gm of acetone-dried porcine posterior pituitaries was 500 mg.

From this type of MSH concentrates from pig glands, Lerner and Lee (1955; Lee and Lerner, 1956) were the first to identify two melanotropins: α-MSH and β-MSH. Later, α-MSH was isolated from equine (Dixon and Li, 1960), bovine (Lo *et al.*, 1961), macacus (Lee *et al.*, 1961), and ovine (Lee *et al.*, 1963) pituitaries. β-MSH was first isolated from porcine glands (Porath *et al.*, 1955; Benley and Purvis, 1956; Geschwind *et al.*, 1956; Geschwind and Li, 1957) and subsequently from bovine (Geschwind *et al.*, 1957b,c), ovine (Lee *et al.*, 1963), equine (Dixon and Li, 1961), and macacus (Lee *et al.*, 1961) glands. From these investigations, it was shown that α-melanotropin consists of 13 amino acids and β-melanotropins of 18 amino acids, except the human β-MSH with 22 amino acids. The isoelectric points of β_b-MSH (b = bovine) and β_p-MSH (p = porcine) were found to be 7.0 and 5.8, respectively (Geschwind *et al.*, 1957c; Geschwind and Li, 1957), whereas the value for α-MSH was 10.5–11.

Isolation of Porcine β-Melanotropin

There are four groups of investigators (Porath *et al.*, 1955; Benley and Purvis, 1956; Lee and Lerner, 1956; Geschwind *et al.*, 1956) who have developed, independently and simultaneously, procedures to obtain β-melanotropin from porcine pituitary glands in highly purified form. Geschwind *et al.* (1956, 1957b) have obtained β-MSH in a form that fulfills various criteria of homogeneity, such as zone electrophoresis, countercurrent distribution, ultracentrifugation, NH_2- and COOH-terminal amino acid analysis, and quantitative data on the constituent amino acids.

The crude MSH concentrate (see above) was fractionated by means of zone electrophoresis on starch in a pyridine–acetate buffer of pH 4.9; the major portion of the MSH activity is concentrated in the main peak. The material recovered from the active peak was submitted to countercurrent distribution in the 2-butanol/0.5% aqueous trichloroacetic acid system through 1100 transfers. The main peak, which contains MSH, was further divided into two fractions and redistributed in the same solvent system for 248 transfers. Both fractions have identical partition coefficients ($K = 0.60$), and each is slightly skewed from the calculated theoretical distribution curve. From 1 kg of acetone-dried posterior lobes of porcine pituitary glands, approximately 175 mg of β_p-melanotropin could be isolated by the procedure just outlined. The purified material before being submitted to countercurrent distribution had an activity of 2×10^{10} units/gm.

Ultracentrifugation of different samples of β-MSH with a synthetic boundary cell gave only a single sedimenting boundary (Geschwind and Li, 1957) with a sedimentation constant of 0.5 S. By equilibrium centrifugation, Porath *et al.* (1955) obtained an approximate molecular weight (MW) of 3000.

Zone electrophoresis of β-MSH on both starch (Geschwind and Li, 1957) and paper (Porath *et al.*, 1955) has shown that it behaves as a homogeneous substance. The isoelectric point of the peptide hormone prepared by Porath *et al*. (1955) in 0.05 *M* phosphate solution was found to be at pH 5.2, whereas that of Geschwind and Li (1957) was reported to be at 5.8, as determined in buffers of 0.1 ionic strength. From the amino acid composition of β-MSH (see below), the isoionic point was calculated to be at pH 5.9, a value in good agreement with the experimentally determined value.

The amino acid analyses of β-MSH give the following 18 amino acid residues in the hormone peptide: $Asp_2Glu_2Ser_1Gly_2Pro_3Met_1Phe_1Tyr_1Lys_2$-$His_1Arg_1Tyr_1$. No amide ammonia is present in the molecule. It is also notable that the common amino acids cystine, threonine, isoleucine, valine, and alanine are all absent. The minimum MW calculated from the empirical formula is 2177, and the theoretical nitrogen content is 16.7%.

III. Isolation of α- and β-Melanotropins from Camel Pituitary Glands

Recently, a new procedure (Li *et al.*, 1975a) was described for the isolation of α- and β-MSH, as well as ACTH, from acid acetone extracts of camel pituitary glands. Acid acetone extract of 500 whole camel pituitaries (650 gm) was obtained as previously described (Li, 1952). The resulting acid acetone powder (20 gm) was dissolved in 1 liter of water at pH 3, and the solution was brought to 0.06 saturation with respect to NaCl. The NaCl precipitate was removed by centrifugation to yield 10 gm of crude prolactin, and the supernatant was brought to saturation with NaCl. The saturated NaCl precipitate was thoroughly dialyzed using the "hollow fiber device" (Bio-Rad, Richmond, California), and the insoluble material was centrifuged off. The clear supernatant was lyophilized and yielded approximately 3.2 gm (designated fraction D).

Fraction D (800 mg) was next submitted to chromatography on a CM cellulose column (1.5 × 45 cm) that had been equilibrated with 0.01 *M* NH_4OAc buffer of pH 4.6. Elution was performed initially with the same buffer. After 3–4 hold-up volumes (4 ml/tube) had been collected, a gradient with respect to pH and concentration was started by introducing 0.1 *M* NH_4OAc buffer of pH 6.7 through a 500-ml mixing flask containing the starting buffer. Later, the gradient was increased by substitution of 0.2 *M* NH_4OAc of pH 6.7 as the solution was flowing into the mixing flask. The chromatographic pattern is shown in Fig. 1. Seven components were obtained, and only components C, D, L, and N were found to contain tryptophan. After lyophilization, yields of the components were C, 130 mg; D, 44 mg; L, 52 mg; and N, 22 mg.

A. β_{C1}-MSH

Forty-four milligrams of component L (see Fig. 1) were submitted to gel filtration on a Sephadex G-25 (fine) column in 0.1 *M* HOAc. As shown in Fig. 2, five peaks were obtained, but only peak C was found to contain tryptophan. The content in peak C was lyophilized, yielded 14 mg, and

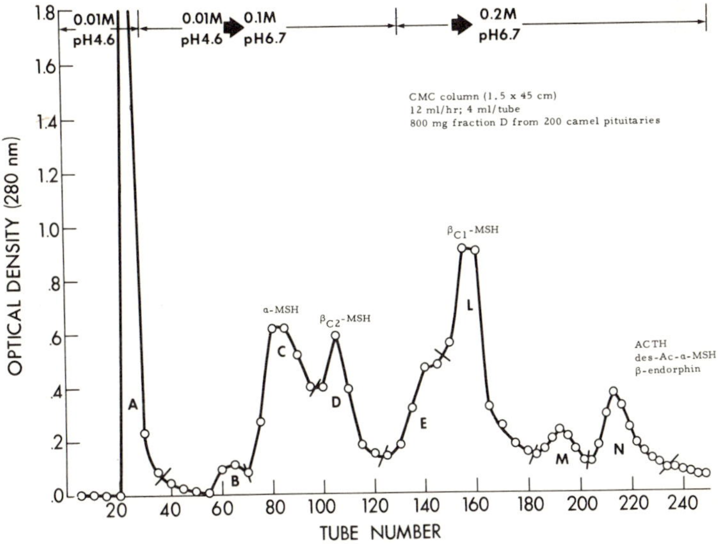

FIG. 1. CM cellulose chromatography of 800 mg fraction D. Column size, 1.5 × 45 cm; flow rate, 12 ml/hour, 4 ml/tube.

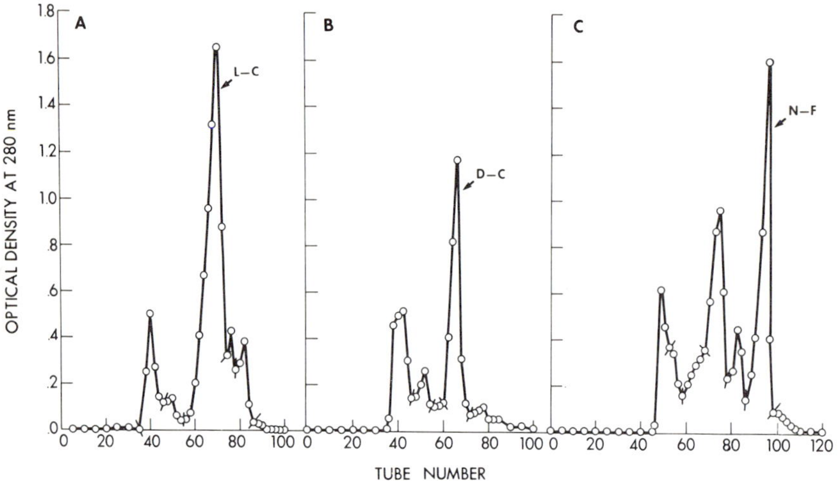

FIG. 2. Gel filtration of components L, D, and N (see Fig. 1) on a Sephadex G-25 (fine) column (3 × 70 cm) in 0.1 *M* HOAc. Flow rate, 9 ml/hour, 3 ml/tube; (A) L, 44 mg; (B) D, 52 mg; and (C) N, 66 mg.

was designated L-C. When L-C was examined in paper electrophoresis at pH 3.7 and 6.7, it was homogeneous with R_f values relative to lysine at 0.54 and 0.32, respectively. Structural data indicate that it is a β-melanotropin.

B. β_{C2}-MSH

Component D (52 mg, Fig. 1) was put on a Sephadex G-25 column in 0.1 *M* HOAc, and the chromatographic pattern may be seen in Fig. 2. The main peak was lyophilized and yielded 9 mg (designated D-C). Paper electrophoresis of D-C gave a single spot at pH 3.7, with an R_f value of 0.19 relative to lysine. Both amino acid and NH_2-terminal sequence analysis are identical with those for β_{C1}-MSH. Additional structural data show that it is another species of β-melanotropin.

C. DES-AC-α-MSH

By similar procedures for the isolation of L-C and D-C, 10 mg of N-F were obtained from 66 mg of component N* (Fig. 1) after gel filtration on Sephadex G-25 in 0.1 *M* HOAc as shown in Fig. 2. The peptide behaved

* ACTH may be isolated from the content in tubes 70–80 (Fig. 2C).

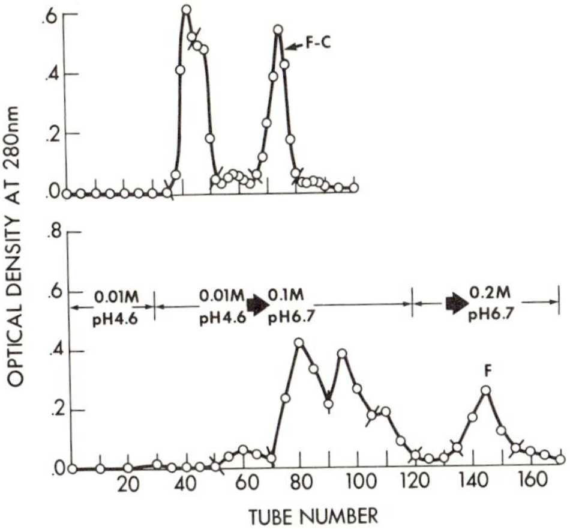

FIG. 3. (Lower) CM cellulose chromatography of 130 mg of material from peak C (Fig. 1). Conditions are the same as Fig. 1. (Upper) Gel filtration of the material in peak F on Sephadex G-25 (fine) column. Same conditions as Fig. 2. Reprinted with permission from Li *et. al.*, (1975a). *Biochemistry* **14,** 947. Copyright by the American Chemical Society.

as a homogeneous substance when tested by paper electrophoresis, as well as by NH_2-terminal and amino acid analyses. Sequence analyses of N-F provide the conclusion that it is deacetylated α-MSH.

D. α-MSH

When 130 mg of component C (Fig. 1) were rechromatographed on the CM cellulose column as shown in Fig. 3, according to the color test, only peak F contained tryptophan. The material in peak F (42 mg) was then lyophilized and submitted to gel filtration on Sephadex G-35 (fine) in 0.1 *M* HOAc. The tryptophan containing component was located in peak F-C (Fig. 3); after lyophilization, it yielded 4 mg. Paper electrophoresis F-C at pH 6.7 indicated that it migrated as a single component with a mobility of 0.43 relative to lysine. No NH_2-terminal residue was detected by the dansyl method. Amino acid analysis of F-C showed that its composition was identical to N-F. Structural data indicate that N-F is α-MSH.

Thus, 16 mg α-MSH, 13 mg deacetylated α-MSH, 67 mg β_{C1}-MSH, and 25 mg β_{C2}-MSH can be isolated in pure form from 500 camel pituitary glands. The same procedure may be employed to obtain melanotropins from glands of other species, including the human pituitary. The melanotropic activities of naturally occurring MSH's from various species are summarized in Table I. It may be noted that α-MSH is the most potent melanotropic agent. Among the β-MSH's, β_{C1}-MSH appears to have the highest potency, which is about one-third of that for α-MSH.

TABLE I—Melanocyte-Stimulating Activity of Various Melanotropins

Hormone	Species	Melanotropic activity[a]
α-MSH	Camel	17.4×10^9
Des-Ac-α-MSH	Camel	2.6×10^9
β-MSH	Human	3.3×10^9
β-MSH	Macacus	4.5×10^9
β-MSH	Equine	1.2×10^9
β-MSH	Porcine	3.8×10^9
β-MSH	Bovine	1.5×10^9
β-MSH	Ovine	1.5×10^9
β_{C1}-MSH	Camel	5.5×10^9
β_{C2}-MSH	Camel	2.9×10^9

[a] Assayed *in vitro;* units/gm.

IV. Structure and Synthesis of α-Melanotropin

The primary structure of porcine α-MSH was first reported by Harris and Lerner (1957). It consists of 13 amino acid residues, and its sequence is identical to the first 13 residues of ACTH, except that the amino group of serine in position 1 is acetylated, and the carboxyl group of valine in position 13 is present as an amide: Ac-Ser-Tyr-Ser-Met-Glu-His-Phe-Arg-Trp-Gly-Lys-Pro-Val-NH_2. It is of interest to note that α-melanotropins from equine (Dixon and Li, 1960), bovine (Lo *et al.,* 1961), macacus (Lee *et al.,* 1961), ovine (Lee *et al.,* 1963), and camel (Li *et al.,* 1975*a*) pituitary glands have the same composition and structure as the porcine hormone (Harris and Lerner, 1957).

Synthesis of α-MSH was first achieved by Guttmann and Boissonnas (1959). Hofman *et al.* (1960) synthesized the glutamine analog of α-MSH. α-MSH was also synthesized by Schwyzer and co-workers (1963a) and Yajima *et al*. (1968a).

α-MSH was also synthesized by the solid-phase method, using phenol resin as a solid support (Blake and Li, 1971). The synthesis followed the standard procedure (Merrifield, 1964), with the exception that the *tert*-butyl protecting group was used for the γ-carboxyl of glutamic acid. This strategy permitted deblocking of the γ-carboxyl before ammonolysis, thus eliminating the danger of side-chain ammonolysis during ammonolytic cleavage of the protected tridecapeptide from the resin. Use of the γ-*tert*-butyl group necessitated the use of the 2-(biphenyl)isopropyloxycarbonyl(Bpoc) group for N^α protection of the five amino terminal residues. The Bpoc group was conveniently removed in 0.05–0.10 *N* HCl in chloroform, a condition which gave minimal hydrolysis of the *tert*-butyl group.

Ammonolysis of the tridecapeptide resin in dimethylformamide at −20° gave the protected tridecapeptide amide. If ammonolysis was carried out at room temperature, the valine residue was extensively racemized. The ammonolytic product was next submitted to reduction with sodium in liquid ammonia and chromatography on CM cellulose. The overall yield of the synthetic α-MSH was 10% on the basis of Boc-valyl resin.

MSH assay of the synthetic product by the *in vitro* procedure showed a potency (2×10^{10} units/gm) equivalent to that of natural α-MSH (see Table I).

V. Synthetic Peptides Related to α-Melanotropin

Synthetic peptides related to α-MSH with a chain length of not more than 13 amino acids are listed in Table II, together with their *in vitro* melanotropic activities. It is seen that the tetrapeptide, His-Phe-Arg-Trp (Eberle *et al.*, 1975), is the smallest peptide known to exhibit melanotropic activity. As the chain length is increased on the amino as well as the carboxyl termini of this tetrapeptide, the melanocyte-stimulating activity increases gradually and approaches that of α-MSH. Thus, His-Phe-Arg-Trp may be considered as the active core of melanotropins.

Yajima *et al.* (1966) synthesized Phe-Arg-Trp-Gly-Lys-Pro-Val-NH_2 and found no melanotropic activity, but an addition of His in this heptapeptide with formyllysine generates a potency of 8.0×10^6 units/gm (Hofmann and Yajima, 1962). This indicates that His is essential for biologic activity.

Replacement of Glu by Gly in Glu-His-Phe-Arg-Trp-Gly does not alter the melanotropic activity (Schnabel and Li, 1960a). Together with the fact that [Gln^5-Lys^{11}(For)]-α-MSH has the same potency of natural α-MSH (Hofmann and Yajima, 1962), it is evident that glutamic acid in position 5 does not play a vital role in the MSH activity.

It was noted that Ser-Tyr-Ser-Met-Gln-His-Phe-Arg has no MSH activity (Hofmann *et al.*, 1957), but an addition of Trp-Gly at the carboxyl terminus to form the decapeptide gives rise to a potency of 2.9×10^6 units/gm (Hofmann and Yajima, 1962). Together with the fact that His-Phe-Arg-Trp-Gly (Schwyzer and Li, 1958) has the same potency as His-Phe-Arg-Trp (Eberle *et al.*, 1975), it appears that Trp in position 9 is essential for activity.

Hofmann *et al.* (1964) reported that the synthetic peptide [4α-

TABLE II—Melanocyte-Stimulating Activity of Synthetic Peptides Related to α-Melanotropin

Synthetic peptide	*In vitro* activity (units/gm)	References[a]
Ac-Ser-Tyr-Ser-Met-Glu-His-Phe-Arg-Trp-Gly-Lys-Pro-Val-NH_2	2.0×10^{10}	1
Ac-Ser-Tyr-Ser-Abu-Gln-His-Phe-Arg-Trp-Gly-Lys-Pro-Val-NH_2	2.6×10^{8}	2
For		
Ac-Ser-Tyr-Ser-Ile-Glu-His-Phe-Arg-Trp-Gly-Lys-Pro-Val-NH_2	1.0×10^{10}	3
Ac-Ser-Tyr-Ser-Leu-Glu-His-Phe-Arg-Trp-Gly-Lys-Pro-Val-NH_2	1.0×10^{10}	3
Ac-Ser-Tyr-Ser-Met-Gln-His-Phe-Arg-Trp-Gly-Lys-Pro-Val-NH_2	2.2×10^{10}	4
For		
Ac-Ser-Tyr-Ser-Met-Gln-His-Phe-Arg-Trp-Gly-Lys-Pro-Val-NH_2	2.0×10^{9}	4
Tos		
Ac-Ser-Met-Glu-His-Phe-Arg-Trp-Gly-Lys-Pro-Val-NH_2	5.0×10^{9}	5
H-Ser-Met-Glu-His-Phe-Arg-Trp-Gly-Lys-Pro-Val-NH_2	1.0×10^{9}	5
H-Glu-His-Phe-Arg-Trp-Gly-Lys-Pro-Val-NH_2	1.4×10^{7}	6
For		
H-His-Phe-Arg-Trp-Gly-Lys-Pro-Val-NH_2	0.8×10^{7}	4
For		
Phe-Arg-Trp-Gly-Lys-Pro-Val-NH_2	0	
H-Lys-Pro-Val-NH_2	1.5×10^{4}	8
Ac-Lys-Pro-Val-NH_2	4×10^{4}	8
H-Gly-Lys-Pro-Val-NH_2	2.5×10^{4}	8
Trp-Gly-Lys-Pro-Val-NH_2	3×10^{5}	8
Ac-Phe-Arg-Trp-Gly-Lys-Pro-Val-NH_2	2.5×10^{6}	8
Ac-Met-Glu-His-Phe-Arg-Trp-Gly-Lys-Pro-Val-NH_2	1.5×10^{9}	8
H-Ser-Tyr-Ser-Met-Gln-His-Phe-Arg-Trp-Gly-OH	2.9×10^{6}	4
H-Ser-Tyr-Ser-Met-Glu-His-Phe-Arg-OH	0	9
H-Ser-Tyr-Ser-Met-Glu-His-Phe-Arg-Trp-Gly-$NHNH_2$	1.0×10^{6}	10
Boc-Ser-Tyr-Ser-Met-Glu-His-Phe-Arg-Trp-Gly-$NHNH_2$	1.0×10^{7}	10
H-Met-Glu-His-Phe-Arg-Trp-Gly-OH	1.4×10^{6}	11
H-Glu-His-Phe-Arg-Trp-Gly-OH	2.0×10^{5}	12
H-Gly-His-Phe-Arg-Trp-Gly-OH	2.0×10^{5}	13
H-His-Phe-Arg-Trp-Gly-OH	3.0×10^{4}	14
H-His-Phe-Arg-Trp-OH	3.6×10^{4}	8
H-Phe-Arg-Trp-Gly-Lys-Pro-Val-NH_2	0	7

[a] 1. Blake and Li (1971); 2. Hofmann *et al.* (1964); 3. Nishimura and Fujino (1972); 4. Hofmann and Yajima (1962); 5. Guttmann and Boissonnas (1961); 6. Yajima *et al.* (1968a); 7. Yajima *et al.* (1966); 8. Eberle *et al.* (1975); 9. Hofmann *et al.* (1957); 10. Li and Hemmasi (1972); 11. Li *et al.* (1961); 12. Li *et al.* (1963); 13. Schnabel and Li (1960a); 14. Schwyzer and Li (1958).

aminobutyric acid, Gln^5]-α-MSH has only 1% of the potency of the parent molecule. Nishimura and Fujino (1972) showed that replacement of Met in position 4 of α-MSH by Leu and Ile does not change significantly the melanotropic activity. These data suggest that Met is not important for the potency of α-MSH.

Modifications of the lysine residue in position 11 of the α-MSH molecule do not always cause loss of melanotropic activity. Formylated lysine analog of α-MSH has the same activity as the natural hormone (Hofmann and Yajima, 1962) but substitution of Lys-11 by N^{ϵ}-Tos-lysine lowers the activity significantly (Hofmann and Yajima, 1962). This is also true if the ϵ-amino function of Lys^{11} in α-MSH is trifluoroacetylated (Stouffer and Watters, 1965).

As already noted in Table I, deacetylated α-MSH is about one-seventh as active as the natural α-MSH. This is also evident from the activities of H-Ser-Tyr-Ser-Met-Gln-His-Phe-Arg-Trp-Gly-$NHNH_2$ and its N^{α}-Boc derivative (Li and Hemmasi, 1972). Apparently, blocking the NH_2-terminal group enhances the melanocyte-stimulating activity. It may also be noted that blocking the α-COOH group at the carboxyl terminus also enhanced the MSH potency (Li and Hemmasi, 1972).

Starting with the pentapeptide, His-Phe-Arg-Trp-Gly, there is a steady increase in melanotropic activity as the NH_2-terminal is built up to the heptapeptide,* Met-Glu-His-Phe-Arg-Trp-Gly. The addition of three more amino acids to the NH_2-terminal does not increase the activity. However, extension of the COOH-terminal by the sequence Lys-Pro-Val-NH_2 results in a thousandfold increase in the activity (see Table II).

Eberle *et al.* (1975) and Eberle and Schwyzer (1975) have recently synthesized a series of peptides related to the COOH-terminal portion of α-melanotropin. Both groups reported that the COOH-terminal tripeptide,† Lys-Pro-Val-NH_2 possesses low but definite melanotropic activity by the *in vitro* assay procedure. The activity increases as the chain length increases at the NH_2-terminus (see Table II). From these and other data, Eberle and Schwyzer (1975) concluded that α-melanotropin possesses two active sites, Met-Glu-His-Phe-Arg-Trp-Gly and Lys-Pro-Val-NH_2 which are capable of independently triggering the hormone receptor responsible for melanin dispersion. From the data summarized in Table II, one of these two active sites is probably His-Phe-Arg-Trp instead of the heptapeptide.

---

* This heptapeptide has been shown to possess *in vitro* corticotropin releasing factor activity (Li *et al.*, 1961; Privat de Garilke *et al.*, 1960; Privat de Garilke and Gros, 1962).

† Medzihradszky and Medzihradszky-Schweiger (1976) reported that the following synthetic tripeptides related to α-MSH possess melanotropic activity: Ac-Lys-Pro-Val-NH_2, 3×10^4 U/gm; H-Glu-His-Phe-OH, 1×10^4 U/gm and H-Arg-Trp-Gly-OMe, 6×10^3 U/gm.

VI. Structure and Synthesis of β-Melanotropins

The structure of porcine β-MSH was first elucidated independently in two laboratories (Geschwind *et al.*, 1956, 1975b; Harris and Roos, 1956). The data obtained by both groups are in complete agreement. These investigators obtained the following amino acid sequence for β-MSH: H-Asp-Glu-Gly-Pro-Tyr-Lys-Met-Glu-His-Phe-Arg-Try-Gly-Ser-Pro-Pro-Lys-Asp-OH.

The two residues of aspartic acid that occur in the peptide occupy the NH_2- and COOH-terminal positions in the chain. Hydrolysis of the hormone peptide with trypsin and chymotrypsin proceeded in accordance with the known specificity of these proteolytic enzymes, with the one exception that the Lys-Asp linkage (positions 17–18) was resistant to cleavage by trypsin.

After the sequence of porcine β-MSH was determined, it was found that the primary structures of the hormone from different species are slightly different [bovine (Geschwind *et al.*, 1957a, 1957c), equine (Dixon and Li, 1961), macacus (Lee *et al.*, 1961), human (Harris and Lerner, 1957; Pickering and Li, 1963), and camel (Li *et al.*, 1975)]. Figure 4 presents the amino acid sequence of known β-melanotropins. All consist of 18 amino acids, except that the human hormone consists of 22 amino acids, and an additional tetrapeptide, Ala-Glu-Lys-Lys, is attached at the NH_2-terminus of monkey β-MSH. Other differences among these β-melanotropins are in positions 2, 6, 8, and 16. The residue in position 2 is either glutamic acid or serine with the exception of camel, where the residue is glycine. One of the camel β-melanotropins has glutamine in position 8 instead of glutamic acid, which occurs in all mammalian hormones. The residue in position 6 is lysine, except that the human and macacus hormones have arginine in this position. Proline is in position 16 for all β-melanotropins, and only the equine hormone has arginine. When the amino acid sequences of all human β-melanotropins are compared (Fig. 4), it is striking that the tetrapeptide His-Phe-Arg-Trp or the pentapeptide His-Phe-Arg-Trp-Gly has been conserved during the evolution from dog fish to man. Indeed, the synthetic His-Phe-Arg-Trp (Eberle *et al.*, 1975) and His-Phe-Arg-Trp-Gly (Schwyzer and Li, 1958) possess melanotropic activity.

Sheep pituitary glands contain two β-melanotropins of bovine and porcine type (Geschwind, 1959; Lee *et al.*, 1963). The biologic activities of both β-melanotropins could be detected in extracts of single sheep pituitaries that had been subjected to zone electrophoresis on starch (Burgers, 1961). Burgers (1961) also demonstrated the existence of components with the mobilities of both these β-melanotropins in extracts of

Human: H-Ala-Glu-Lys-Lys-Asp-Glu-Gly-Pro-Tyr-Arg-Met-Glu-His-Phe-Arg-Trp-Gly-Ser-Pro-Pro-Lys-Asp-OH

Macacus: H-Asp-Glu-Gly-Pro-Tyr-Arg-Met-Glu-His-Phe-Arg-Trp-Gly-Ser-Pro-Pro-Lys-Asp-OH

Porcine: H-Asp-Glu-Gly-Pro-Tyr-Lys-Met-Glu-His-Phe-Arg-Trp-Gly-Ser-Pro-Pro-Lys-Asp-OH

Equine: H-Asp-Glu-Gly-Pro-Tyr-Lys-Met-Glu-His-Phe-Arg-Trp-Gly-Ser-Pro-Arg-Lys-Asp-OH

Bovine: H-Asp-Ser-Gly-Pro-Tyr-Lys-Met-Glu-His-Phe-Arg-Trp-Gly-Ser-Pro-Pro-Lys-Asp-OH

Camel: H-Asp-Gly-Gly-Pro-Tyr-Lys-Met-Glu-His-Phe-Arg-Trp-Gly-Ser-Pro-Pro-Lys-Asp-OH

Camel: H-Asp-Gly-Gly-Pro-Tyr-Lys-Met-Gln-His-Phe-Arg-Trp-Gly-Ser-Pro-Pro-Lys-Asp-OH
1 5 10 15 18

FIG. 4. Amino acid sequences of β-melanotropins from various species.

single bovine and porcine glands. In their study of monkey melanotropins Lee *et al*. (1961), noted the existence of a small amount of [Ser[2]] β_m-MSH (m = monkey) in addition to β_m-MSH (see Fig. 4).

Attempts to synthesize β-MSH (Schwyzer *et al.,* 1959) proved futile until the advent of protecting groups derived from *tert*-butanol. Schwyzer and co-workers (1963b) succeeded in synthesizing an octadecapeptide corresponding to the structure of bovine β-MSH.

In the earlier attempt to synthesize porcine β-MSH, Schwyzer *et al.* (1959) used the methyl group for blocking the β-carboxyl groups of aspartic acid residues and the tosyl residues for masking the ε-amino groups of lysine residues. When the protecting groups were removed by saponification followed by treatment with sodium in liquid ammonia, a mixture of products resulted. In the new successful synthesis (Schwyzer *et al.,* 1963b), all the protecting groups could be removed by treatment with trifluoroacetic acid.

Monkey and human β-MSH were synthesized by Yajima and his co-workers (1968a, 1969b, 1970). Human β-MSH was also synthesized by Rittel (1968). Wang *et al*. (1973) reported the synthesis of human and monkey β-MSH by the solid-phase method. Recently, using the solid-phase procedure, Li *et al*. (1975b) synthesized camel β_{C1}-MSH, with a final yield of 25%, based on starting N^{α}-Boc-Bzl-Asp resin.

Reaction of the tetramethylammonium salt of N^{α}-Boc-(β-Bzl) Asp with chloromethylated polymer gave N^{α}-Boc-(β-Bzl)Asp resin, which was then subjected to the procedure for solid-phase peptide synthesis. Removal of the N^{α}-Boc protecting group was carried out by treatment for 15 minutes in 50% trifluoroacetic acid in dichloromethane. Coupling of Boc–amino acid was achieved with dicyclohexylcarbodiimide along with use of the following side-chain protecting groups: serine and aspartic acid, benzyl; lysine and tyrosine, *o*-bromobenzyloxycarbonyl; arginine, tosyl; histidine, Boc, and tryptophan, formyl. The glutamine residue was introduced using its *p*-nitrophenyl ester. The finished peptide was cleaved from the resin, and all protecting groups were removed with liquid HF, with the exception of the formyl group. Preliminary purification was carried out by gel filtration on Sephadex G-10 and G-25. For deformylation, the material recovered from Sephadex G-25 was treated with 1 *M* NH_4HCO_3, pH 9.0, at 25° for 24 hours. The deformylated product was submitted to chromatography on CM cellulose; the material from the main peak was further purified by partition chromatography on Sephadex G-25. The peptide recovered from the main peak in this step was shown to be the desired product. When the synthetic product and the natural hormone were subjected to partition chromatography on the same column, they behaved identically, with an R_f value of 0.22. Gel filtration on Sephadex G-25 of both natural and synthetic hormones gave a single peak with $V_s/V_0 = 1.45$. The behavior of the synthetic product on paper electrophoresis at pH 3.7 and pH 6.9 was identical with that of the natural hormone. Polyacrylamide gel electrophoresis at pH 4.5 of both natural and synthetic hormones showed a single band for each with the same mobility. Amino acid analysis of acid and enzymic hydrolyzates of the synthetic product gave values in agreement with the data obtained with the natural hormone. Electrophoretic patterns of tryptic and chymotryptic digests and synthetic β_{C1}-MSH were also identical. Values for optical rotation of synthetic and natural hormones did not differ significantly. Table III presents the biologic data for the synthetic and natural β_{C1}-MSH. It is evident that both

TABLE III—Biologic Activities of Synthetic β_{C1}-MSH

	Synthetic		Natural	
Bioassay	Dose (ng)	Response	Dose (ng)	Response
Melanotropic activity[a]	3	52.8 ± 3.6	3	53.7 ± 5.4
	9	66.5 ± 0.6	9	67.0 ± 0.4
Lipolytic activity[b]	17	1.60 ± 0.2	17	1.75 ± 0.03
	51	3.98 ± 0.3	51	4.26 ± 0

[a] Melanotropic activity expressed as percent decrease in reflectance. Five skins used for each assay. Values expressed in mean ± SE. The potency of the synthetic β_{C1}-MSH is computed to be 95% of the natural hormone with 95% confidence limit of 51–160 and λ of 0.2.

[b] Lipolytic activity expressed in μmole glycerol production/gm cells/hour. Triplicate determinations with values expressed in mean ± SE. The synthetic β_{C1}-MSH is computed to be 91% of the natural hormone with confidence limit of 74–111 and λ of 0.04.

the melanocyte-stimulating and lipolytic activities of the synthetic product are identical with those exhibited by natural β_{C1}-MSH.

VII. Structure–Activity Relationships of β-MSH by Synthetic Approach

The relationship between chain length and biologic activity of β-melanotropin has been investigated by Yajima *et al.* (1966, 1967b, 1969b). As noted in Table IV, the heptapeptide Phe-Arg-Trp-Gly-Ser-Pro-Pro has no melanotropic activity. However, additions of amino acids on either end of the heptapeptide increase the MSH potency. Further elongation of the decapeptide chain to the pentadecapeptide Pro-Tyr-Arg-Met-Gln-His-Phe-Arg-Trp-Gly-Ser-Pro-Pro-Lys(F)-Asp increases the potency comparable to that of α-MSH. Apparently, addition of acidic peptide units, Asp-Gly-Gly or Ala-Glu-Lys-Lys-Asp-Glu-Gly, to this pentadecapeptide to form monkey and human β-MSH, respectively, causes a lowering of the melanotropic activity.

Recently, Lemaire *et al.* (1977) investigated the importance of residues in positions 2, 8, 10, and 12 in β_{C1}-MSH (see Fig. 4) by solid-phase synthesis of these analogs. The melanotropic and lipolytic activities of synthetic β-melanotropins and analogs are summarized in Tables V and VI. It may be noted in Table V that replacement of Gln^8 of β_{C1}-MSH by Arg induced

TABLE IV—Synthetic Peptides Related to β-Melanotropin

<table>
<tr><th>Synthetic peptides</th><th>In vitro activity (units/gm)</th><th>References[a]</th></tr>
<tr><td>H-Phe-Arg-Trp-Gly-Ser-Pro-Pro-OH</td><td>0</td><td>1</td></tr>
<tr><td>F
|
H-His-Phe-Arg-Trp-Gly-Ser-Pro-Pro-Lys-Asp-OH</td><td>2.4×10^6</td><td>2</td></tr>
<tr><td>F
|
H-Glu-His-Phe-Arg-Trp-Gly-Ser-Pro-Pro-Lys-Asp-OH</td><td>6.0×10^6</td><td>3</td></tr>
<tr><td>F
|
H-Arg-Met-Glu-His-Phe-Arg-Trp-Gly-Ser-Pro-Pro-Lys-Asp-OH</td><td>1.8×10^8</td><td>3</td></tr>
<tr><td>F
|
H-Pro-Tyr-Arg-Met-Glu-His-Phe-Arg-Trp-Gly-Ser-Pro-Pro-Lys-Asp-OH</td><td>2.2×10^{10}</td><td>3</td></tr>
</table>

[a] 1. Yajima *et al.* (1966); 2. Yajima *et al.* (1967b); 3. Yajima *et al.* (1969a).

TABLE V—Melanotropic Activity of Synthetic β-Melanotropins and Analogs

			Potency		
Melanotropin	Dose (ng)	Response[a]	%	95% Confidence limit	λ
β_{C1}-MSH	3	32.7 ± 3.6			
	9	63.5 ± 1.1			
[Arg^8]-β_{C1}-MSH	6	17.1 ± 2.8	10.5[b]	5.2–16.5	0.12
	18	24.6 ± 1.7			
CHO | [Trp^{12}]-β_{C1}-MSH	6	32.8 ± 6.2	39.7[b]	29.4–53.6	0.12
	18	52.4 ± 1.3			
β_{C1}-MSH	6	62 ± 1.7			
	18	71 ± 0.4			
[Gly^{10}]-β_{C1}-MSH	6	5.5 ± 1.7	0.8[b]	0.01–3.8	0.20
	18	7.8 ± 0.8			
[Phe^{12}]-β_{C1}-MSH	6	26.2 ± 3.4	28[b]	6.8–123	0.27
	18	38.2 ± 5.4			
Natural β_b-MSH	2.3	29.1 ± 3.7			
	6.9	44.6 ± 2.0			
β_b-MSH	2.7	30.1 ± 3.7	120.2[c]	81.2–186.2	0.16
	8.1	49.6 ± 1.6			
β_p-MSH	2.6	49.6 ± 3.4	355.6[c]	251.5–604.0	0.12
	7.8	69.8 ± 1.1			

[a] MSH activity expressed as percent decrease in reflectance. Five skins used for each assay. Values in mean ± SE.

[b] Compared with synthetic β_{C1}-MSH.

[c] Compared with natural β_b-MSH.

a large decrease in its melanotropic activity to only 10.5%. The ineffectiveness of [Gly^{10}]-β_{C1}-MSH in stimulating frog skin darkening was also observed. However, [formyl-Trp^{12}]-β_{C1}-MSH retained 39.7% of the melanotropic activity of the parent peptide, and replacement of Trp^{12} of β_{C1}-MSH by Phe also gave a fairly active compound (28% compared with the activity of the parent peptide). Finally, β_p-MSH was three times more active than β_b-MSH with regard to melanotropic activity, as noted in Table I. The only difference between these two molecules is that residue number 2 of β_b-MSH is Ser, instead of Glu, for β_p-MSH (Fig. 4).

As shown in Table VI, the lipolytic activity of synthetic β_{C1}-MSH was found to be 2.2 times higher than that of β_b-MSH. Replacement of Gln^8 of β_{C1}-MSH by Arg lowered the activity of 34.2% of the original value for β_{C1}-MSH. Changes in positions 10 and 12 of β_{C1}-MSH appeared to have a more dramatic effect on lipolytic activity than changes in positions 8. [Formyl-Trp^{12}]-β_{C1}-MSH retained only 10.2% of the activity of the parent peptide, while [Gly^{10}]-and [Phe^{12}]-β_{C1}-MSH had no lipolytic activity. Alteration in position 2 of β-melanotropin did not seem to modify its lipolytic activity, β_b-MSH being as active as β_p-MSH.

Alteration in Trp^{12} of β_{C1}-MSH greatly affected its lipolytic activity (Table VI). An alteration of Trp^{12} as small as its formylation drops the lipolytic activity of β_{C1}-MSH to 10% of its original value, and we must not exclude the possibility that this low level of activity of [formyl-Trp^{12}]-β_{C1}-MSH might be due to some β_{C1}-MSH arising from deformylation during either the purification or the lipolytic assay. Finally, replacement of Trp^{12} by Phe completely destroyed the lipolytic activity (Table VI). On the other hand, Phe^{12}-β_{C1}-MSH retained 28% of the melanotropic activity of

TABLE VI—Lipolytic Activity of Synthetic Melanotropins and Analogs

			Potency		
Synthetic	Dose	Response[a] (ng)	%	95% Confidence limit	λ
β_{C1}-MSH	37	2.94 ± 0.03			
	111	3.60 ± 0.15			
β_b-MSH	37	1.78 ± 0.05	40.2[b]	26.3–55.2	0.09
	111	2.96 ± 0.15			
[Arg^8]-β_{C1}-MSH	37	1.73 ± 0.10	34.2[b]	21.9–46.7	0.09
	111	3.12 ± 0.15			
CHO | [Trp^{12}]-β_{C1}-MSH	37	1.09 ± 0.23	10.2[b]	0.1–23.5	0.17
	111	2.05 ± 0.19			
[Phe^{12}]-β_{C1}-MSH	1100	1.29 ± 0.09	0.006[b]	0–0.034	0.26
	3300	1.63 ± 0.29			
[Gly^{10}]-β_{C1}-MSH	1100	0.19 ± 0.04	0.001[b]	0–0.00012	0.16
	3300	0.37 ± 0.05			
Natural β_b-MSH	22	1.38 ± 0.1			
	66	3.76 ± 0.1			
β_b-MSH	22	1.18 ± 0.1	95.5[c]	93.3–125.9	0.03
	66	3.61 ± 0.1			
β_p-MSH	22	1.62 ± 0.1	102.4[c]	85.1–107.2	0.05
	66	3.49 ± 0.1			

[a] Micromole of glycerol production per gram of cells per hour. Determinations in triplicate. Values in mean ± SE.

[b] Compared with β_{C1}-MSH.

[c] Compared with natural β_b-MSH.

the parent peptide (Table V). Thus, the structural requirements of these two activities in the β-melanotropin molecule are different.

The structural requirements for melanotropic activity of β-melanotropins showed other differences from those for lipolytic activity. The melanotropic activity of β_{C1}-MSH was dependent upon the integrity of Gln^8, while the lipolytic activity depended more on that of Trp^{12} (Tables V and VI). It may also be noted that changes at position 2 of β-MSH affect the melanotropic activity while the lipolytic activity is untouched. Therefore, the postulate (Ramachandran, 1973) that the melanotropic action of peptides related to ACTH should correlate with their ability to stimulate lipolysis in rabbit fat cells may not be entirely true for β-MSH.

The findings that $[Gly^{10}]$-β_{C1}-MSH has neither lipolytic nor melanotropic activities pinpoint the importance of Phe^{10} of β_{C1}-MSH. With regard to previous results, which indicated that replacement of Phe^7 of ACTH-(1–24) by Leu gives a compound with 20% of the steroidogenic activity of the parent peptide (Fujino *et al.*, 1971), one might speculate that the hydrophobicity of the side chain in this position is involved in its biologic activity.

VIII. Dogfish Melanotropins

The existence of melanotropins in the nonmammalian vertebrate pituitary glands has been reported by several investigators (Burgers, 1961, 1963; Love and Pickering, 1969). The isolation and structure of an α-MSH from an elasmobranch, the dogfish *(Squalus acanthias),* were first achieved by Lowry and Chadwick (1970) who showed that 10 of its 11 residues are the same as 10 of the 13 residues of mammalian α-MSH:

H-Ser-Met-Glu-His-Phe-Arg-Trp-Gly-Pro-Met-NH_2

Unlike the mammalian hormone, however, none of it was found to be N^{α}-acetylated. The melanotropic activity of the dogfish α-MSH is about one-hundredth of mammalian α-MSH potency. Watanabe and Yajima (1974) reported the synthesis of this nonmammalian vertebrate α-MSH and showed that the Zn complex of the synthetic peptide had higher melanotropic activity than that of the natural hormone.

The presence of β-MSH in the pituitary of the dogfish *(Scyliorhinus canicula)* was first indicated by the experiment of Love and Pickering (1972). These investigators (1974) were subsequently able to isolate 7 mg active peptide from 4000 dogfish pituitary glands. The isolated material contained two active peptides by paper electrophoresis, but they appeared to have the same amino acid composition, probably differing by the presence of a side-chain amide. Sequence analysis of the peptide established the primary structure related to β-MSH:

H-Asp-Gly-Ile-Asp-Tyr-Lys-Met-Gly-His-Phe-Arg-Trp-Gly-Ala-Pro-Met-Asp-Lys-OH

Bennett *et al*. (1974) reported also the isolation and structure of a β-MSH type peptide from the spiny dogfish *(Squalus acanthias):*

H-Asp-Gly-Asp-Asp-Tyr-Lys-Phe-Gly-His-Phe-Arg-Trp-Ser-Val-Pro-Leu-OH

Figure 5 compares the structures of the dogfish melanotropins with those from mammalian species. The occurrence of tetrapeptide His-Phe-Arg-Trp-Gly in all species is striking. This tetrapeptide has been conserved during the evolution from dogfish to man (see Fig. 4). Indeed, the synthesis of His-Phe-Arg-Trp (Eberle *et al.,* 1975) possesses melanotropic activity (see Table II). It may also be noted that the greatest difference between dogfish β-melanotropins and all mammalian β-MSH (see Table VI) is the presence of glycine in position 8 as all β-melanotropins have Glu in this position. However, this may not be so surprising as Schnabel and Li (1960a) found that the synthetic hexapeptide Gly-His-Phe-Arg-Trp-Gly was just as active as Glu-His-Phe-Arg-Trp-Gly. The other interesting difference in *Scyliorhinus* β-MSH is the presence of two methionine residues; the second residue is in the position analogous to that found in *Squalus* α-MSH (Lowry and Chadwick, 1970). It is also interesting that the COOH-terminal sequence -Asp-Lys-OH is inverted as compared with the mammalian β-melanotropins.

IX. Various Studies on β-Melanotropin

Porcine β-MSH was examined as acceptor in the reaction catalyzed by arginyl–tRNA transferase (Soffer, 1975). Briefly, the reaction mixture for arginylation of β-MSH (10 ml) contained 50 m*M* Tris–HCl (pH 9.0), 0.1 *M*

Scyliorhinus caniculus:	H-Asp-Gly-Ile-Asp-Tyr-Lys-Met-Gly-His-Phe-Arg-Trp-Gly-Ala-Pro-Met-Asp-Lys-OH
Squalus acanthias:	H-Asp-Gly-Asp-Asp-Tyr-Lys-Phe-Gly-His-Phe-Arg-Trp-Ser-Val-Pro-Leu-OH
Squalus acanthias:	H-Ser-Met-Glu-His-Phe-Arg-Trp-Gly-Lys-Pro-Met-NH_2
Squalus acanthias:	H-Ser-Met-Glu-His-Phe-Arg-Trp-Gly-Lys-Pro-Met-OH
Squalus acanthias:	H-Tyr-Ser-Met-Glu-His-Phe-Arg-Trp-Gly-Lys-Pro-Met-NH_2

FIG. 5. Amino acid sequences of dogfish melanotropins.

2-mercaptoethanol, 0.15 *M* KCl, 10 m*M* magnesium acetate, 3 m*M* ATP, 0.025% sodium azide, 0.32 m*M* [^{14}C]arginine (15 μCi-μmole), 0.12 m*M* β-MSH, and 10 units of arginyl–tRNA synthetase, 5 mg of *Escherichia coli* B tRNA and 2 units of arginyl–tRNA transferase per milliliter, respectively. Incubation was performed at 37° for 18 hours. Analysis by paper electrophoresis indicated that 1040 nmole of arginine were converted to a peptide-dependent product with an R_{arg} of 0.55. It was found that β_p-MSH and its arginylated derivative had identical activities in the frog skin assay.

The secondary structure of β_p-MSH has been studied with circular dichroism and infrared spectroscopy methods (Makarov *et al.,* 1975). A left-handed poly-L-proline II-type helix has been shown in aqueous solution. It becomes more stable on cooling in the solution, and its content lowers in 60% ethanol. Relative humidity and H-D exchange effects on the hormone films show that the twisted β-form and the extended poly-L-proline II type helix are present.

X. Inactivation and Activation

After the purified β-MSH obtained from zone electrophoresis on starch had been submitted to countercurrent distribution, it was observed that the pure product had undergone partial inactivation (Geschwind and Li, 1957). It has not been ascertainable whether this inactivation is due to "denaturation" of the β-MSH molecule or to a chemical modification of the peptide in the course of the distribution at 20°. However, it was found that a new component of low activity, possessing a partition coefficient of 0.35, appeared when the material was redistributed in the same solvent system. It is possible that the methionine residue has been oxidized to methionine sulfoxide (Lo *et al.,* 1961).

Lee and Lerner (1956) have investigated the stability of their preparation of α-MSH and found that it could be kept at a temperature of −17° in a nitrogen or oxygen atmosphere, or *in vacuo,* for a period of 19 days, with some, but not marked, loss of activity. Table VII shows that storage for 50 days in the air and *in vacuo* also resulted in a decrease of potency. These workers also noted that the hormone is relatively unstable in an oxygen atmosphere at room temperature. The crude MSH concentrate was quite stable for many months in the air at room temperature (I. I. Geschwind and C. H. Li, unpublished observations). It has been demonstrated that the activity of β-MSH is destroyed by peroxide, but not by reduction with potassium borohydride (Dixon, 1956). The peroxide-treated β-MSH can be regenerated with thioglycolate, in a similar fashion to what has been

TABLE VII—Stability of α-MSH[a]

Atmosphere	Storage temperature	Storage interval (days)	Potency after storage (units/mg × 10^6)	Original potency remaining (%)
Vacuum	−17°	19	7.7	59
Nitrogen	−17°	19	7.0	54
Oxygen	−17°	19	7.4	57
H_2S	−17°	19	2.0	15
Oxygen	20°–25°	19	1.4	11
Vacuum	−17°	50	2.5	16
Air	−17°	50	3.5	22

[a] Taken from Lee and Lerner (1956).

observed with ACTH. Landgrebe and Mitchell (1954) showed that solutions of purified melanotropin in 0.25% acetic acid are stable at room temperature for at least 4 months if heated in small ampules in a boiling water bath for 1 minute and sealed while still hot.

As early as 1922, Hogben and Winton showed that melanocyte-stimulating activity in an extract of posterior pituitaries is destroyed by digestion with trypsin, but not with pepsin. These observations have now been confirmed with the pure β-MSH, and it has been found that the hormone is readily inactivated by chymotryptic digestion (I. I. Geschwind and C. H. Li, unpublished data).

One of the remarkable properties of the melanotropins was first reported by Hogben and Gordon (1930), who observed that the addition of NaOH (final concentration 1.35 *M*) to a posterior lobe extract abolished the vasopressor effect but increased the melanocyte-stimulating effect. This striking effect of alkali on the activity of melanotropin has been repeatedly confirmed by various investigators. For example, according to Abramowitz (1937), the melanocyte-stimulating effect of the pituitary of the *Fundulus* is increased about 25-fold by being boiled in 0.1 *M* NaOH. Waring and Landgrebe (1950) summarized the effect as follows: "Caustic soda treatment of unfractioned posterior-lobe extracts modified their melanophore-excitant properties in at least two ways: (a) the melanophore-expanding potency is increased, as judged by peak melanophore index attained; (b) there is an increased duration of response when submaximal doses are injected." The former effect was called "potentiation" and the latter "protection" or "prolongation" (Landgrebe and Waring, 1950). Experiments with isolated skin of dogfish also show that alkali–heat treatment of extracts result in both potentiation and protection. In fact, these phenomena have been used by some investigators to differentiate the bovine from the porcine melanotropin (Benley and Purvis, 1956; Landgrebe and Mitchell, 1954) and to establish the nonidentity of the melanotropins and the corticotropins (Geschwind *et al.,* 1952; Morris, 1952).

Geschwind and Li (1964) studied effects of alkaline–heat treatment with β_p-MSH and β_b-MSH in detail. When β_p-MSH or β_b-MSH in 0.1 *M* NaOH was heated at 100° C for 10 minutes, conversion of arginine to ornithine occurred, and there was a loss of aspartic acid, serine, proline, and lysine. The amounts of arginine, histidine, methionine, and phenylalanine found by microbiologic analyses of a treated preparation are significantly lower than those found by the DNP procedure (Levy, 1954).

Cleavage of a peptide bond in β-MSH molecules also occurs when the hormone is submitted to sodium hydroxide–heat treatment. This is evident from amino acid analyses, which are consistent with a loss of the COOH-terminal sequence Ser-Pro-Pro-Lys-Asp-OH (see Fig. 4) from approximately 40% of the molecules of treated β_b-MSH. Apparently, the peptide bond Gly 13-Ser 14 is quite sensitive to alkaline hydrolysis. That this is the bond that is cleaved was confirmed by digestion of treated MSH with carboxypeptidase, which released glycine from its C-terminal position and tryptophan from its position adjacent to glycine, in addition to aspartic acid, which is the COOH-terminal residue of the parent molecule.

Primarily on the basis of an increased resistance on the part of treated ACTH concentrate to enzymatic digestion, Raben (1955) suggested that racemization was responsible for the prolongation phenomenon. Microbiologic analyses of treated β_b-MSH (Geschwind and Li, 1964) as shown in Table VIII appear to confirm Raben's suggestion. In addition, enzymatic digestion of treated ACTH (Pickering and Li, 1964) and α-MSH (Lee *et al.,* 1963), has revealed racemization of arginine, histidine, and methionine in these hormones. The racemization of phenylalanine is comparatively extensive in the melanotropins, which contain but one residue per mole, but not in ACTH, which contains three (Li, 1962). Tyrosine has been reported to be racemized in α-MSH (Lee *et al.,* 1963), although to a lesser extent than any of the aforementioned amino acids. It is tempting to suggest that all the racemization of phenylalanine in ACTH occurs in the single residue of the heptapeptide core, and, consequently, that racemization is extensive only for those residues in the core. One of the other two phenylalanine residues is C-terminal, and racemization of this residue would be expected to be inhibited because of the presence of the terminal COOH group on this amino acid (Neuberger, 1948). Supporting this contention is the finding (Pickering and Li, 1964) that carboxypeptidase released phenylalanine from treated ACTH as readily as it did from

TABLE VIII—Composition of Alkali–Heat Treated β_b-MSH as Determined by Dinitrophenyl (DNP) and Microbiologic Amino Acid Analyses

Amino acid	No. of residues per mole MSH: Control		NaOH–heat treated		% D-isomer in NaOH-treated MSH
	DNP	Microbiol.	DNP	Microbiol.	
Glu	1.05	—[a]	1.08	—[a]	
Asp	1.99	2.10	**1.57**[b]	1.69	
Ser[c]	2.06	—[d]	**1.60**	—[d]	
Gly	2.09	—	2.01	—	
Pro	3.00	2.90	**2.18**	2.24[d]	
Met	0.96	0.97	0.98	0.60[e]	39
Phe	1.01	1.11	0.97	0.56	42
Tyr	1.02	0.93	0.89	0.84	
His	0.95	1.02	0.96	0.71	26
Lys	2.01	2.10	**1.43**	1.39	
Arg	0.98	0.89	0.72	0.37	49
Orn	—	—	0.27	—	

[a] No specific organism for L-Glu available.
[b] Bold face values are significantly different from control dinitrophenyl amino acid analyses.
[c] Values are corrected for 15% hydrolysis.
[d] High blank made assay unreliable.
[e] Values in italics are significantly different from dinitrophenyl amino acid analyses of the same hydrolyzate.

a control preparation. The other three amino acids of the core are glycine, glutamic acid, and tryptophan. In explanation of the increased resistance of treated α-MSH (Lee *et al.*, 1963) to proteolysis by trypsin and chymotrypsin, it was found that the arginine, phenylalanine, tryptophan, tyrosine, and lysine in the molecule were extensively racemized. However, the results with ACTH (Pickering and Li, 1963) show only 5% racemization for lysine and 6% for tyrosine.

The partial conversion of arginine to ornithine was first observed by I. I. Geschwind and C. H. Li (unpublished data) after treatment of the synthetic peptides H-His-Phe-Arg-Tyr-Gly-OH and H-Glu-His-Phe-Arg-Try-Gly-OH. This transformation was also found in additional experiments with ACTH (Pickering and Li, 1964).

Interestingly, a synthetic pentapeptide containing both D-Phe and L-Orn [L-His-D-Phe-L-Orn-L-Try-Gly (Li *et al.*, 1960)] showed prolongation of activity without having to be heated in alkali. Li *et al*. (1960) found that the synthetic peptide L-His-L-Phe-L-Orn-L-Tyr-Gly, even though it contains an ornithine residue, is of itself not protected, but can be protected by heating in alkali. From a consideration of these observations, together with the findings of Geschwind and Li (1964), it may be concluded that racemization alone is responsible for the prolongation effect of alkali–heat treatment of melanotropically active hormone.

NaOH treatment of the pentapeptide His-Phe-Arg-Trp-Gly and its melanotropic activity were investigated by Hano *et al.* (1966). Treatment of the synthetic pentapeptide with 0.1 *M* NaOH at 100° for 10 minutes gave rise to 40-fold increase in the MSH activity, as revealed by the *in vitro* frog skin assay. Chemical and enzymic examination of the treated peptide showed that one-quarter of Arg was converted to ornithine and four amino acid residues, namely, His, Phe, Arg, Trp were racemized. Potentiation of the melanotropic activity was observed, and no prolongation effects could be detected. Table IX gives the melanotropic activity of various stereoisomers of H-His-Phe-Arg-Trp-Gly-OH. It is interesting that the pentapeptide-containing D-amino acids were not active, and D-Phe and D-Trp analogs of the pentapeptide exhibited approximately 160 and 20 times higher activity than that of the all-L-pentapeptides, respectively.

XI. Concluding Remarks

The role of melanotropins in pigmentary control is well established in amphibians, fish, and reptiles. Their functions in mammals are not clearly defined, although it has been demonstrated that they are involved in visual adaptation (Jores, 1933; Hanaoka, 1953), behavioral activity (Ferrari *et*

TABLE IX—Synthetic Stereoisomers of His-Phe-Arg-Trp-Gly and Their Melanotropic Activities

His-	Phe-	Arg-	Trp-	units/gm	Reference[a]
L	L	L	L	3.0×10^4	1
D	L	L	L	0	2
L	D	L	L	3.3×10^5	3
L	L	D	L	0	4
L	L	L	D	1.0×10^5	2
D	L	D	L	0	5
L	D	L	D	1.0×10^6	5
D	D	D	D	0	6

[a] 1. Schwyzer and Li (1958); 2. Yajima and Kubo (1965a,b); 3. Schnabel and Li (1960a); 4. Yajima *et al.* (1966); 5. Yajima *et al.* (1967b); 6. Yajima and Kubo (1965a).

al., 1963; Ferrari, 1958; De Wied *et al.*, 1975; Sandman *et al.*, 1971, 1972), radioprotection (Sakamoto and Prasad, 1967), thyroid function (Bowers *et al.*, 1964), sebaceous gland activity (Thody and Shuster, 1975; Ebling *et al.*, 1975), and skin darkening (McGuire and Lerner, 1963; Geschwind *et al.*, 1972). Recently, Plotnikoff and Kastin (1976) showed that α-melanotropin potentiates the behavioral effects of dopamine, but not serotonin, and slightly reduces footshock-induced fighting in susceptible mice. Melanotropins, no doubt, exert direct actions on the central nervous system in addition to their endocrine functions. Future investigations on structure–function relationships of melanotropins will enable us to localize active sites in these molecules for their various activities.

Acknowledgment

I thank the following colleagues for their contributions in these studies on melanotropins: I. I. Geschwind, L. Barnafi, J. S. Dixon, D. Chung, B. T. Pickering, J. Blake, K. T. Wang, D. Yamashiro, and S. Lemaire. I also thank the National Institutes of Health and the Allen-Geffen Fund for support during the course of these studies and the writing of this review.

References

Abe, K., Island, D. P., Liddle, G. W., Fleischer, N., and Nicholson, W. E. (1967a). *J. Clin. Endocrinol. Metab.* **27**, 46.

Abe, K., Nicholson, W. E., Liddle, G. W., Island, D. P., and Orth, D. N. (1967b). *J. Clin. Invest.* **46**, 1609.

Abramowitz, A. A. (1937). *Biol. Bull.* **73**, 134.

Allen, B. M. (1916). *Science* **44**, 755.

Allen, B. M. (1920). *Science* **52**, 274.

Barth, R. (1960). *Acta Endocrinol. (Copenhagen)* **35**, 454.

Benley, B. J., and Purvis, J. L. (1956). *Biochem. J.* **62**, 588.

Bennett, H., Lowry, P. J., McMartin, C., and Scott, P. A. (1974). *Biochem. J.* **141**, 439.

Bjorklund, A., Meurling, P., Nilsson, G., and Nobin, A. (1972). *J. Endocrinol.* **53**, 161.

Blake, J., and Li, C. H. (1971). *Int. J. Protein Res.* **3**, 185.

Bowers, C. Y., Redding, T. W., and Schally, A. V. (1964). *Endocrinology* **74**, 559.

Burgers, A. C. J. (1961). *Endocrinology* **68**, 698.

Burgers, A. C. J. (1963). *Ann. N.Y. Acad. Sci.* **100**, 669.

Cehovic, G. (1962). *C. R. Acad. Sci. (Paris)* **254**, 1872.

Courrier, R., and Cehovic, G. (1960). *C. R. Acad. Sci. (Paris)* **251**, 832.

De Wied, D. (1966). *Proc. Soc. Exp. Biol. Med.* **122**, 28.

De Wied, D., and Bohns, B. (1966). *Nature (London)* **212**, 1484.

De Wied, D., Witter, A., and Greven, H. M. (1975). *Biochem. Pharmacol.* **24**, 1463.

Dixon, H. B. F. (1956). *Biochim. Biophys. Acta* **19**, 392.

Dixon, H. B. F. (1960). *Biochim. Biophys. Acta* **37**, 38.

Dixon, J. S., and Li, C. H. (1960). *J. Am. Chem. Soc.* **82**, 4569.

Dixon, J. S., and Li, C. H. (1961). *Gen. Comp. Endocrinol.* **1,** 161.
Donnadien, M., and Sevaux, D. (1974). *Biomedicine* **19,** 272.
Eberle, A., and Schwyzer, R. (1975). *Helv. Chim. Acta* **58,** 1528.
Eberle, A., Fauchere, J.-L., Tesser, G. I., and Schwyzer, R. (1975). *Helv. Chim. Acta* **58,** 2106.
Ebling, F. J., Ebling, E., Randall, V., and Skinner, J. (1975). *J. Endocrinol.* **66,** 407.
Ferrari, W. (1958). *Nature (London)* **181,** 925.
Ferrari, W., Gossa, G. L., and Vargui, L. (1963). *Ann. N.Y. Acad. Sci.* **104,** 330.
Frieden, E. H., Fishbein, J. W., and Hisaw, F. L. (1948). *Arch. Biochem.* **17,** 183.
Fujino, M., Hatanaka, C., Nishimura, O., and Shinagawa, S. (1971). *Chem. Pharm. Bull.* **19,** 1075.
Geiling, E. M. K. (1935). *Bull. Johns Hopkins Hosp.* **57,** 123.
Geiling, E. M. K. (1942). *Harvey Lect.* **37,** 269.
Geschwind, I. I. (1959). *In* "Comparative Endocrinology" (A. Gorbman, ed.), p. 421. Wiley, New York.
Geschwind, I. I., and Huseby, R. A. (1966). *Endocrinology* **79,** 97.
Geschwind, I. I., and Huseby, R. A. (1969). *Prog. Endocrinol., Proc. Int. Congr. Endocrinol., 3rd, 1968* Excerpta Med. Found. Int. Congr. Ser. No. 157, p. 70.
Geschwind, I. I., and Li, C. H. (1957). *J. Am. Chem. Soc.* **79,** 615.
Geschwind, I. I., and Li, C. H. (1964). *Arch. Biochem. Biophys.* **106,** 200.
Geschwind, I. I., Reinhardt, W. O., and Li, C. H. (1952). *Nature (London)* **169,** 1061.
Geschwind, I. I., Li, C. H., and Barnafi, L. (1956). *J. Am. Chem. Soc.* **78,** 620.
Geschwind, I. I., Li, C. H., and Barnafi, L. (1957a). *J. Am. Chem. Soc.* **79,** 620.
Geschwind, I. I., Li, C. H., and Barnafi, L. (1957b). *J. Am. Chem. Soc.* **79,** 1003.
Geschwind, I. I., Li, C. H., and Barnafi, L. (1957c). *J. Am. Chem. Soc.* **79,** 6394.
Geschwind, I. I., Huseby, R. A., and Nishioka, R. (1972). *Recent Prog. Horm. Res.* **28,** 91.
Guttmann, S., and Boissonnas, R. A. (1959). *Helv. Chim. Acta* **42,** 1257.
Guttmann, S., and Boissonnas, R. A. (1961). *Experientia* **17,** 265.
Hadley, M. E., and Bagnara, J. T. (1975). *In* "Trends in Comparative Endocrinology" (E. J. W. Barrington, ed.), p. 81. Am. Soc. Zoologists.
Hanaoka, T. (1951). *Jpn. J. Physiol.* **2,** 9.
Hanaoka, T. (1953). *Nature (London)* **172,** 866.
Hano, K., Koida, M., Yajima, H., Kubo, K., and Oshima, T. (1966). *Biochim. Biophys. Acta* **115,** 337.
Harris, J. I., and Lerner, A. B. (1957). *Nature (London)* **179,** 1346.
Harris, J. I., and Roos, P. (1956). *Nature (London)* **178,** 90.
Hofmann, K., and Yajima, H. (1962). *Recent Prog. Horm. Res.* **18,** 41.
Hofmann, K., Thompson, T. A., and Schwartz, E. T. (1957). *J. Am. Chem. Soc.* **79,** 6087.
Hofmann, K., Yajima, H., and Schwartz, E. T. (1960). *J. Am. Chem. Soc.* **82,** 3732.
Hofmann, K., Rosenthaler, J., Wells, R. D., and Yajima, H. (1964). *J. Am. Chem. Soc.* **86,** 4991.
Hogben, L. T., and Gordon, C. (1930). *J. Exp. Biol.* **7,** 286.
Hogben, L. T., and Slome, D. (1931). *Proc. R. Soc. London, Ser. B* **108,** 10.
Hogben, L. T., and Wintin, F. R. (1922). *Biochem. J.* **16,** 619.
Howe, A. (1973). *J. Endocrinol.* **59,** 385.
Jores, A. (1933). *Klin. Wochenschr.* **12,** 1599.
Jores, A., and Glogner O. (1933). *Z. Gesamte Exp. Med.* **91,** 91.
Kamm, O. Aldrich, T. B., Grote, I. W., Rowe, L. W., and Bugbee, E. P. (1928). *J. Am. Chem. Soc.* **50,** 573.
Kleinholz, L. H., and Rahn, H. (1940). *Anat. Rec.* **76,** 157.

Krivoy, W. A., and Guillemin, R. (1961). *Endocrinology* **69,** 170.
Landgrebe, F. W., and Mitchell, G. M. (1954). *Q. J. Exp. Physiol. Cogn. Med. Sci.* **39,** 11.
Landgrebe, F. W., and Waring, H. (1950). *In* "Hormone Assay" (C. W. Emmens, ed.), p. 141. Academic Press, New York.
Landgrebe, F. W., Ketterer, B., and Waring, H. (1955). *Hormones* **3,** 421.
Lee, T. H., and Lerner, A. B. (1956). *J. Biol. Chem.* **221,** 943.
Lee, T. H., Lerner, A. B., and Buethner-Janusch, V. (1961). *J. Biol. Chem.* **236,** 1390.
Lee, T. H., Lerner, A. B., and Buethner-Janusch, V. (1963). *Biochim. Biophys. Acta* **71,** 706.
Lemaire, S., Yamashiro, D., Rao, A. J., and Li, C. H. (1977). *J. Med. Chem.* **20,** 155.
Lerner, A. B., and Lee, T. H. (1955). *J. Am. Chem. Soc.* **77,** 1066.
Lerner, A. B., and McGuire, J. S. (1961). *Nature (London)* **189,** 176.
Lerner, A. B., and Takahashi, Y. (1956). *Recent Prog. Horm. Res.* **12,** 303.
Lerner, A. B., and Wright, M. R. (1960). *Methods Biochem. Anal.* **8,** 295.
Lerner, A. B., Shizume, K., and Bunding, I. (1954). *J. Clin. Endocrinol. Metab.* **14,** 1463.
Levy, A. L. (1954). *Nature (London)* **174,** 126.
Li, C. H. (1952). *Acta Endocrinol. (Copenhagen)* **10,** 255.
Li, C. H. (1957). *Adv. Protein Chem.* **12,** 269.
Li, C. H. (1962). *Surv. Biol. Prog.* **4,** 93.
Li, C. H., and Hemmasi, B. (1972). *J. Med. Chem.* **15,** 697.
Li, C. H., Schnabel, E., and Chung, D. (1960). *J. Am. Chem. Soc.* **82,** 2062.
Li, C. H., Schnabel, E., Chung, D., and Lo, T. B. (1961). *Nature (London)* **189,** 143.
Li, C. H., Gorup, B., Chung, D., and Ramachandran, J. (1963). *J. Org. Chem.* **28,** 178.
Li, C. H., Danho, W. O., Chung, D., and Rao, A. J. (1975a). *Biochemistry* **14,** 947.
Li, C. H., Yamashiro, D., and Lemaire, S. (1975b). *Biochemistry* **14,** 953.
Lo, T. B., Dixon, J. S., and Li, C. H. (1961). *Biochim. Biophys. Acta* **53,** 584.
Long, J. M., Krivoy, W. A., and Guillemin, R. (1961). *Endocrinology* **69,** 176.
Love, R. M., and Pickering, B. T. (1969). *Gen. Comp. Endocrinol.* **13,** 425.
Love, R. M., and Pickering, B. T. (1972). *Gen. Comp. Endocrinol.* **18,** 604.
Love, R. M., and Pickering, B. T. (1974). *Gen. Comp. Endocrinol.* **24,** 398.
Lowry, P. J., and Chadwick, A. (1970). *Biochem. J.* **118,** 713.
McGuire, J., McGill, R., Leeman, S., and Goodfriend, T. (1965). *J. Clin. Invest.* **44,** 1672.
McGuire, J. S., and Lerner, A. B. (1963). *Ann. N.Y. Acad. Sci.* **100,** 622.
Makarov, A. A., Esipova, N. G., Pankov, Y. A., Lobachev, V. M., and Grishkovsky, B. A. (1975). *Biochem. Biophys. Res. Commun.* **67,** 1378.
Medzihradszky, K., and Medzihradszky-Schweiger, H. (1976). *FEBS Lett* **67,** 45.
Merrifield, R. B. (1964). *Biochemistry* **3,** 1385.
Morris, C. J. O. R. (1952). *Lancet* No. 6720, 1210.
Mussio Fournier, J. C., Morato-Manero, J., and Fischer, J. T. (1936). *An. Fac. Med., Univ. Repub., Montevideo* **21** (8–9).
Mussio Fournier, J. C., Cervino, J. M., and Conti, V. (1943). *J. Clin. Endocrinol.* **3,** 353.
Neuberger, A. (1948). *Adv. Protein Chem.* **4,** 297.
Nishimura, O., and Fujino, M. (1972). *J. Takeda Res. Lab.* **31,** 293.
Pickering, B. T., and Li, C. H. (1963). *Biochim. Biophys. Acta* **74,** 156.
Pickering, B. T., and Li, C. H. (1964). *Arch. Biochem. Biophys.* **104,** 119.
Plotnikoff, N. P., and Kastin, A. J. (1976). *Life Sci.* **18,** 1217.
Porath, J., Roos, P., Landgrebe, F. W., and Mitchell, G. M. (1955). *Biochim. Biophys. Acta* **17,** 598.
Privat de Garilhe, M., and Gros, C. (1962). *Experientia* **18,** 92.
Privat de Garilhe, M., Gros, C., Porath, J., and Lindner, E. B. (1960). *Experientia* **16,** 414.
Raben, M. S. (1955). *Abstr. 37th Annu. Meet. Am. Endocr. Soc.* p.20

Ramachandran, J. (1970). *Biochem. Biophys. Res. Commun.* **41,** 353.

Ramachandran, J. (1973). *In* "Hormonal Proteins and Peptides" (C. H. Li, ed.), Vol. 2, p. 1. Academic Press, New York.

Rittel, W. (1968). *Adv. Exp. Med. Biol.* **2,** 35.

Roth, A. (1932). *Z. Pathol. Anat.* **54,** 234.

Rust, C. C. (1965). *Gen. Comp. Endocrinol.* **5,** 222.

Sakamoto, A. (1966). *Nature (London)* **211,** 1370.

Sakamoto, A., and Prasad, K. N. (1967). *Int. J. Radiat. Biol.* **12,** 97.

Sandman, C. A., Kastin, A. J., and Schally, A. V. (1971). *Physiol. Behav.* **6,** 45.

Sandman, C. A., Miller, L. H., Kastin, A. J., and Schally, A. V. (1972). *J. Comp. Physiol. Psychol.* **80,** 54.

Schnabel, E., and Li, C. H. (1960a). *J. Biol. Chem.* **235,** 2010.

Schnabel, E., and Li, C. H. (1960b). *Biochim. Biophys. Acta* **97,** 596.

Schwyzer, R., and Li, C. H. (1958). *Nature (London)* **182,** 1669.

Schwyzer, R., Kappeler, H., Iselin, B., Rittel, W., and Zuber, H. (1959). *Helv. Chim. Acta* **42,** 1702.

Schwyzer, R., Costopanagiotes, A., and Sieber, P. (1963a). *Helv. Chim. Acta* **46,** 870.

Schwyzer, R., Iselin, B., Kappeler, H., Riniker, B., Rittle, W., and Zuber, H. (1963b). *Helv. Chim. Acta* **46,** 1975.

Shizume, K., Lerner, A. B., and Fitzpatrick, R. B. (1954). *Endocrinology* **54,** 553.

Smith, P. E. (1916). *J. Endocrinol.* **25,** 249.

Smith, P. E. (1919). *Proc. Soc. Exp. Biol. Med.* **16,** 74.

Smith, P. E., and Smith, I. P. (1923). *Anat. Rec.* **25,** 150.

Snell, R. S. (1962). *J. Endocrinol.* **25,** 249.

Soffer, R. L. (1975). *J. Biol. Chem.* **250,** 2626.

Steelman, S. L., Kelley, T. L., Norgello, H., and Wever, G. F. (1956). *Proc. Soc. Exp. Biol. Med.* **92,** 392.

Stouffer, J. E., and Watters, J. A., Jr. (1965). *Biochim. Biophys. Acta* **104,** 214–217.

Swingle, W. W. (1921). *J. Exp. Zool.* **34,** 119.

Thing, E. (1952). *Acta Endocrinol. (Copenhagen)* **10,** 295.

Thing, E. (1953a). *Acta Endocrinol. (Copenhagen)* **11,** 363.

Thing. E. (1953b). *Acta Endocrinol. (Copenhagen)* **13,** 29.

Thody, A. J., and Shuster, S. (1973). *Nature (London)* **245,** 207.

Thody, A. J., and Shuster, S. (1975). *J. Endocrinol.* **64,** 503.

Thody, A. J., Cooper, M. F., Bowden, P. E., Meddis, D., and Shuster, S. (1976). *J. Endocrinol.* **71,** 279.

Tilders, F. J. H., van Delft, A. M. C., and Smelik, P. G. (1975). *J. Endocrinol.* **66,** 165.

Trendelenburg, P. (1924). *Klin. Wochenschr.* **3,** 777.

Usategni, R., Oliver, C., Vandry, H., Lombardi, G., Rozenberg, I., and Monroe, A. M. (1976). *Endocrinology* **98,** 189.

Van Dyke, H. B. (1936). "The Physiology and Pharmacology of the Pituitary Body," Vol. I. Univ. of Chicago Press, Chicago, Illinois.

Wang, K. T., Blake, J., and Li, C. H. (1973). *Int. J. Pept. Protein Res.* **5,** 33.

Waring, H., and Landgrebe, F. W. (1950). *Hormones* **2,** 506.

Watanabe, H., and Yajima, H. (1974). *Chem. Pharm. Bull.* **22,** 1894.

Wright, P. L. (1946). *Anat. Rec.* **96,** 44.

Yajima, H., and Kubo, K. (1965a). *Biochim. Biophys. Acta* **97,** 596.

Yajima, H., and Kubo, K. (1965b). *J. Am. Chem. Soc.* **87,** 2039.

Yajima, H., Okada, Y., Oschimura, T., and Lande, S. (1966). *Chem. Pharm. Bull.* **14,** 707.

Yajima, H., Okada, Y., Kimomura, Y., and Seto, E. (1967a). *Chem. Pharm. Bull.* **15,** 270.

Yajima, H., Kubo, K., and Kimomura, Y. (1967b). *Chem. Pharm. Bull.* **15,** 504.
Yajima, H., Okada, Y., Kimomura, Y., and Minami, H. (1968a). *J. Am. Chem. Soc.* **90,** 527.
Yajima, H., Kawasaki, K., Okada, Y., Minami, H., Kubo, K., and Yamashita, I. (1968b). *Chem. Pharm. Bull.* **16,** 919.
Yajima, H., Okada, Y., Kawatami, H., and Mizokami, N. (1969a). *Chem. Pharm. Bull.* **17,** 1229.
Yajima, H., Kawasaki, K., Minami, H., Kawatami, H., Mizokami, N., and Okada, Y. (1969b). *Biochim. Biophys. Acta* **175,** 228.
Yajima, H., Kawasaki, K., Minami, H., Kawatami, H., Mizokami, N., Kiso, Y., and Tamura, F. (1970). *Chem. Pharm. Bull.* **18,** 1394.
Zondek, B., and Krohn, H. (1932). *Klin. Wochenschr.* **11,** 405.

2

β-Endorphin: A New Biologically Active Peptide from Pituitary Glands

CHOH HAO LI

I. Introduction*

It has been postulated for many years that opiates must bind to receptors in nerve cells in order to produce their characteristic responses (Bec-

* Abbreviations: β-LPH, β-lipotropin; β_h-LPH, human β-lipotropin; β-EP, β-endorphin (subscripts c, h, and s denote camel, human, and sheep β-endorphin, respectively); MSH, melanotropin; CM cellulose, carboxymethylcellulose; icv, intraventricularly; iv, intravenously; ip, intraperitoneally; sc, subcutaneously; GH, somatotropin, growth hormone; RIA, radioimmunoassay; JOR, jaw-opening reflex, 5-HTP, 5-hydroxytryptophan; MED, minimal effective dose, UTP, uridine triphosphate, TFE, trifluoroethanol; TFA, trifluoroacetic acid.

kett, 1959). In 1971, Goldstein *et al.* showed that pharmacologically relevant opiate receptor binding should be stereospecific. They incubated mouse brain homogenate with ^{3}H-labeled levorphanol in the presence of an 100-fold excess of unlabeled dextrorphan or levorphanol. Stereospecific binding was defined as that portion of the binding that was blocked by levorphanol, but not by dextrorphan. These investigators (Goldstein *et al.*, 1971) reported that the stereospecific binding of levorphanol represents only 2% of the total binding. Subsequently, Simon *et al.* (1973), Terenius (1973), and Pert and Snyder (1973) described independently similar modifications of the Goldstein procedure to show that stereospecific opiate binding in rat brain homogenates represented the major portion of total association of drug with tissue. Pert *et al.* (1975) reported the occurrence of opiate receptors in the central nervous systems of all vertebrates including the most primitive fish. From these investigations, it was speculated that the brain may contain a hitherto unidentified substance, which normally acts as the endogenous activator of the opiate receptors.

In 1975, Hughes reported a material in mammalian brain extracts that acts similarly to morphine in inhibiting electrically induced contraction of smooth muscle. Terenius and Wahlström (1975) and Pasternak *et al.* (1975) described the existence of a morphinelike substance in extracts of calf, rabbit, and rat brain. The compound has a molecular weight (MW) of approximately 1000 and is inactivated by carboxypeptidase A and B, as well as by leucine aminopeptidase, and, to a lesser extent, by chymotrypsin, but not by trypsin. Evidence for the existence of a similar substance in human cerebrospinal fluid was also reported by Terenius and Wahlström (1975). Subsequently, Hughes *et al.* (1975) isolated, characterized, and synthesized two naturally occurring pentapeptides in pig brain: H-Tyr-Gly-Gly-Phe-Met-OH (Met-enkephalin) and H-Tyr-Gly-Gly-Phe-Leu-OH (leu-enkephalin) in a ratio of approximately 3 : 1. Both peptides acted like morphine on the guinea pig ileum and mouse vas deferens preparations. Met-enkephalin is about 20 times more potent than morphine in the receptor assay. Leu-enkephalin is somewhat less potent than the methionine analog. Goldstein *et al.* (1976) synthesized a heptapeptide (H-Tyr-Gly-Gly-Gly-Lys-Met-Gly-OH) based purely on theoretical grounds with an opioid potency of approximately 1/5000 of normorphine. Recently Simantov and Snyder (1976a,b) identified leu-enkephalin and met-enkephalin from bovine brain extracts and found that bovine brain contains four times as much leu-enkephalin as met-enkephalin. These investigators (Simantov and Snyder, 1976b) also suggested that leu-enkephalin may be a purer agonist than met-enkephalin.

When administered through permanently indwelling cannulae in the lateral ventricles of rats, met-enkephalin and leu-enkephalin induce a profound analgesia *in vivo,* with very short duration, that is fully reversible by naloxone (Belluzzi *et al.,* 1976; Büscher *et al.,* 1976). When injected intravenously (iv) in the mouse, the maximum effect of morphine occurred after 15 minutes (ED_{50} = 2.0 mg/kg), whereas met-enkephalin exhibited a transient effect at very high doses (ED_{50} = 170 mg/kg), analgesic activity being detected only within 15 seconds of administration (Büscher *et al.,* 1976).

Figure 1 shows that met-enkephalin is a peptide fragment of β-lipotropin (β-LPH) corresponding to residues 61–65. β-LPH was first discovered and isolated from sheep pituitary glands in 1964 (Li, 1964; Birk and Li, 1964). It has also been obtained in highly purified form from bovine (Lohmar and Li, 1967), porcine (Gráf and Cseh, 1968; Gilardeau and Chrétien, 1970; Yudeau and Pankov, 1970), and human (Cseh *et al.*, 1968; Scott and Lowry, 1974; Li and Chung, 1976b; Chrétien *et al.*, 1976c) pituitaries. The complete amino acid sequences of ovine (Li *et al.*, 1965, 1966; Gráf and Li, 1973), porcine (Gráf *et al.*, 1971; Gilardeau and Chrétien, 1972; Pankov and Yudeau, 1972), and human (Li and Chung, 1976b) hormones have been proposed. From a comparison of the structures of various lipotropins (see Fig. 1), it is evident that the sequence of COOH-terminal 56 residues is surprisingly homologous, whereas the amino acid sequence at the NH_2-terminal exhibits considerable variability.

II. Isolation of β-Endorphin

During the course of isolation of melanotropins from camel pituitary glands (Li *et al.*, 1975), we were unable to find the existence of β-LPH, but obtained an untriakontapeptide (Li and Chung, 1976a) that has an amino acid sequence identical to the COOH-terminal 31 residues of ovine lipotropin [β_s-LPH-(61–91)] (see Fig. 1). The peptide possesses very low lipotropic activity but significant opiate activity (Li and Chung, 1976a), as displayed in a preparation of guinea pig ileum and in the opiate receptor-binding assay (Cox *et al.,* 1976). This untriakontapeptide was designated β-endorphin (β-EP) (Li and Chung, 1976a). Bradbury *et al*. (1976a,b) and Gráf *et al*. (1976a) also obtained a similar untriakontapeptide from porcine pituitary glands with opiate activity.

Two laboratories (Chrétien *et al.,* 1976b; Li *et al.,* 1976a) described independently the isolation of human β-EP by the procedure previously described for the ovine hormone (Li *et al.,* 1965, 1966). One thousand frozen whole human pituitary glands were finely ground and extracted with 2 liters of acid–acetone solution which was prepared by mixing 250 ml water, 1700 ml acetone, and 50 ml concentrated HCl. After vigorous

	5 10
Human:	H-Glu-Leu-Thr-Gly-Gln-Arg-Leu-Arg-Gln-Gly-
Ovine:	H-Glu-Leu-Thr-Gly-Glu-Arg-Leu-Glu-Gln-Ala-
Porcine:	H-Glu-Leu-Ala-Gly-Ala-Pro-Pro-Glu-Pro-Ala-
	15 20
	Asp-Gly-Pro-Asn-Ala-Gly-Ala-Asn-Asp-Gly-
	Arg-Gly-Pro-Glu-Ala-Gln-Ala-Glu-Ser-Ala-
	Arg-Asp-Pro-Glu-Ala-Pro-Ala-Glu-Gly-Ala-
	25 30
	Glu-Gly-Pro-Asn-Ala-Leu-Glu-His-Ser-Leu-
	Ala-Ala-Arg-Ala-Glu-Leu-Glu-Tyr-Gly-Leu-
	Ala-Ala-Arg-Ala-Glu-Leu-Glu-His-Gly-Leu-
	35 40
	Leu-Ala-Asp-Leu-Val-Ala-Ala-Glu-Lys-Lys-
	Val-Ala-Glu-Ala-Glu-Ala-Ala-Glu-Lys-Lys-
	Val-Ala-Glu-Ala-Gln-Ala-Ala-Glu-Lys-Lys-
	45 50
	Asp-Glu-Gly-Pro-Tyr-Arg-Met-Glu-His-Phe-
	Asp-Ser-Gly-Pro-Tyr-Lys-Met-Glu-His-Phe-
	Asp-Glu-Gly-Pro-Tyr-Lys-Met-Glu-His-Phe-
	55 60
	Arg-Trp-Gly-Ser-Pro-Pro-Lys-Asp-Lys-Arg-
	Arg-Trp-Gly-Ser-Pro-Pro-Lys-Asp-Lys-Arg-
	Arg-Trp-Gly-Ser-Pro-Pro-Lys-Asp-Lys-Arg-
	65 70
	Tyr-Gly-Gly-Phe-Met-Thr-Ser-Glu-Lys-Ser-
	Tyr-Gly-Gly-Phe-Met-Thr-Ser-Glu-Lys-Ser-
	Tyr-Gly-Gly-Phe-Met-Thr-Ser-Glu-Lys-Ser-
	75 80
	Gln-Thr-Pro-Leu-Val-Thr-Leu-Phe-Lys-Asn-
	Gln-Thr-Pro-Leu-Val-Thr-Leu-Phe-Lys-Asn-
	Gln-Thr-Pro-Leu-Val-Thr-Leu-Phe-Lys-Asn-
	85 91
	Ala-Ile-Ile-Lys-Asn-Ala-Tyr-Lys-Lys-Gly-Glu-OH
	Ala-Ile-Ile-Lys-Asn-Ala-His-Lys-Lys-Gly-Gln-OH
	Ala-Ile-Val-Lys-Asn-Ala-His-Lys-Lys-Gly-Gln-OH

FIG. 1. Amino acid sequences of human, porcine, and ovine β-lipotropin.

stirring for 1 hour, the mixture was centrifuged and the residue reextracted with 1 liter of 80% acetone. After removal of the residue by centrifugation, the clear supernatant was poured into 15 liters of cold acetone. The precipitate formed was dried in vacuum after repeated washing with acetone. The product was designated as acid–acetone powder (AAP), and the yield from 1000 glands averaged 12 gm.

The AAP (12 gm) was next dissolved in 500 ml H_2O and adjusted to pH 3.0. A saturated NaCl solution (32 ml) was added drop by drop with constant stirring; the precipitate formed was centrifuged off and saved for the isolation of somatotropin–prolactin. The supernatant was brought to saturation with solid NaCl. The saturated NaCl precipitate was thoroughly dialyzed using the "hollow fiber device" (Bio-Rad, Richmond, California), and the insoluble material was centrifuged off. The clear supernatant was lyophilized and yielded approximately 1.2 gm (designated Fraction D).

Fraction D (500 mg) was next submitted to chromatography on a CM cellulose column (1.5 × 45 cm) that had been equilibrated with 0.01 *M* NH_4OAc buffer of pH 4.6. Elution was performed initially with the same buffer. After three–four hold-up volumes (4 ml/tube) had been collected, a gradient with respect to pH and concentration was started by introducing 0.1 *M* NH_4OAc buffer of pH 6.7 through a 500-ml mixing flask containing the starting buffer. Later, the gradient was increased by substitution of 0.2 *M* NH_4OAc of pH 6.7 as the solution flowed into the mixing flask. Thirteen components were obtained and submitted to paper electrophoresis on Whatman No. 3MM paper in pyridine–HOAc buffer of pH 3.7 (pyridine–HOAc–H_2O, 4 : 40 : 1150, v/v) for 2 hours at 400 V; synthetic β_h–LPH^{61-91} was used as reference (see Fig. 2). It was found that only component L″ (33 mg from two CMC columns) had a spot which migrated identically to the synthetic material. Gel filtration of L″ on Sephadex G-25 column (3 × 70 cm) in 0.1 *M* HOAc gave two fractions, and the retarded fraction (6 mg) was further purified by paper electrophoresis. The main component from the electrophoretogram was eluted and yielded 2.5 mg (designated L″2-1). Chemical and biologic studies of L″2-1 showed that it is human β-endorphin (β_h-EP) (Li *et al.,* 1976a). Thus, only 3 mg of β_h-EP were obtained from 1000 fresh-frozen human glands. Interestingly, 50 mg of β_h-LPH could be isolated from the same extracts (Li and Chung, 1976b).

III. Primary Structure

Amino acid composition of β_h-EP was found to be: $Lys_{4.6}Asp_{2.2}Thr_{2.8}Ser_{2.0}Glu_{3.2}Pro_{1.0}Gly_{2.7}Ala_{2.3}Val_{0.8}Met_{0.8}Ile_{0.9}Leu_{1.9}Tyr_{1.6}Phe_{1.8}$.

The tryptic map of β_h-EP gave six spots and one faint spot as shown in Fig. 3. Amino acid compositions of the spots were: T1, Lys; T2, $Lys_{0.9}Glu_{1.2}Gly_{0.9}$; T3, $Lys_{0.8}Asp_{1.1}Ala_{1.1}Tyr_{1.0}$; T4, $Glu_{1.1}Gly_{0.8}$; T5, $Lys_{1.0}Asp_{1.0}Ala_{1.1}Ile_{1.9}$ (72-hour hydrolysis); T6, $Lys_{1.1}Thr_{0.9}Ser_{0.9}Glu_{1.1}Gly_{1.8}Met_{0.7}Tyr_{0.9}Phe_{1.1}$; T6A, $Lys_{1.1}Thr_{1.0}Ser_{1.1}Glu_{1.3}Gly_{1.9}Met_{0.7}Tyr_{0.9}Phe_{1.0}$; T7, $Lys_{1.0}Thr_{2.0}Ser_{0.8}Glu_{1.2}Pro_{1.0}Val_{0.9}Leu_{2.1}Phe_{1.0}$. From these data and the sequence of β_c-EP (Li and Chung, 1976a), β_h-EP may be derived from

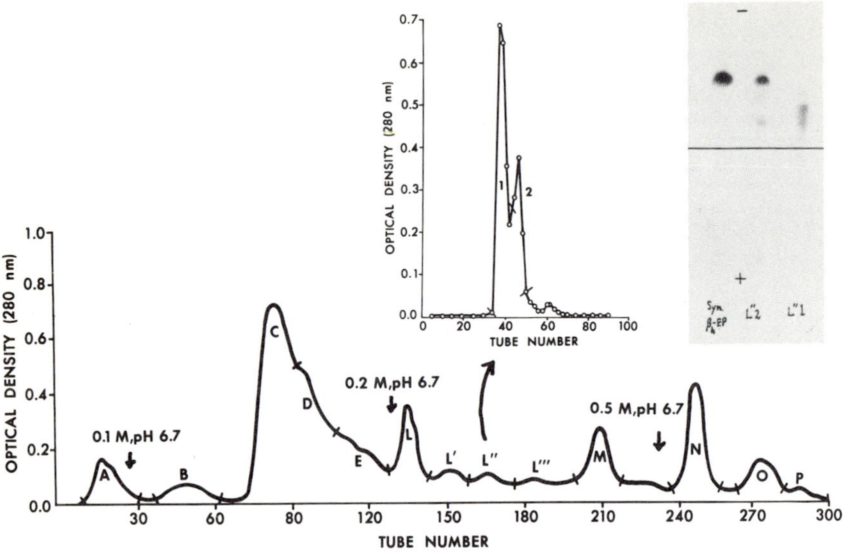

FIG. 2. Isolation procedures for β_h-EP (see text). Bottom, CM cellulose chromatographic pattern of Fraction D; Upper left, gel filtration on Sephadex G-25 of L″; Upper right, paper electrophoresis of L″2 and L″1.

the COOH-terminal 31-amino acid fragment (see Fig. 1) of β_h-LPH (Li and Chung, 1976b). It should be noted that the faint spot 6A (see Fig. 3) is most probably the methionine sulfoxide analog of spot 6, as they both had identical amino acid composition in their acid hydrolyzates.

In order to ascertain that β_h-EP is, indeed, the COOH-terminal fragment of β_h-LPH, it was submitted to comparison with the synthetic β_h-LPH$^{61-91}$. They were found to behave identically in paper electrophoresis and thin-layer chromatography. Tryptic maps of the synthetic product and β_h-EP are also identical. Figure 3 presents the amino acid sequence of β_h-EP.

IV. Synthesis

Both camel (Li *et al.*, 1976a) and human (Li *et al.*, 1977a) β-endorphins have been synthesized by the solid-phase method (Merrifield, 1963). Synthesis of the protected peptide corresponding to the sequence of β_h-EP was performed on brominated styrene–1% divinylbenzene polymer (Merrifield, 1963).

Chloromethylated styrene–1% divinylbenzene (5.10 gm, Lab Systems

LS-601, 0.9 mmole Cl/gm) was stirred in CCl_4 (40 ml) for 10 minutes. Iodine (165 mg), and a solution of bromine (8 ml) in CCl_4 (17 ml) were added; the mixture was stirred for 20 hours at 24° in the dark. The resin was filtered off and washed with 150 ml each of dioxane, H_2O, 1 *M* $NaHCO_3$, H_2O, DMF, H_2O, and methanol yield 8.432 gm (weight gain, 66%; theoretical weight gain for monobromination of every aromatic ring, 71%).

The tetramethylammonium salt of Boc(Bzl)Glu-OH was allowed to react with brominated resin in DMF for 21 hours at 25° and worked up as previously described (Yamashiro and Li, 1973). Removal of the Boc group and admine determination (Gisin, 1972) gave 0.28 mmole/gm.

Boc(Bzl)Glu-bromo polymer was carried through the same schedule for synthesis described previously (Yamashiro *et al.*, 1976) with the following

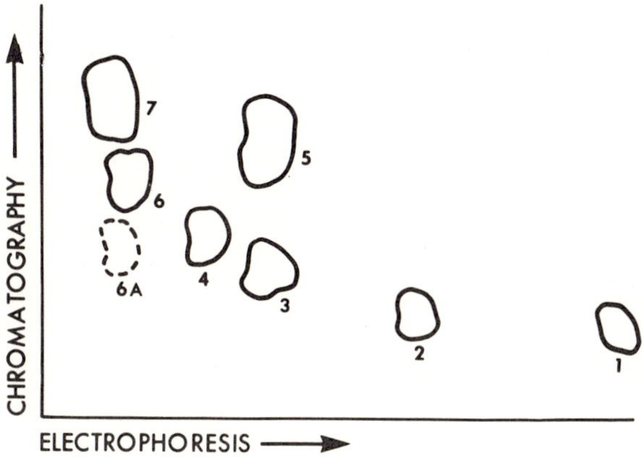

Two-dimensional chromatography-electrophoresis pattern of
the tryptic digest of β_h-endorphin

----

1 5 10
H-Tyr-Gly-Gly-Phe-Met-Thr-Ser-Glu-Lys-Ser-
|←—— T6 ——→|←—

15 20
Gln-Thr-Pro-Leu-Val-Thr-Leu-Phe-Lys-Asn-
—— T7 ——→|←—

25 31
Ala- Ile- Ile- Lys-Asn-Ala-Tyr-Lys-Lys-Gly-Glu-OH
—T5 ——→|←— T3 ——→|←— T2 ——→|

Proposed amino acid sequence of β_h-endorphin

FIG. 3. Upper, two-dimensional chromatographic–electrophoretic pattern of the tryptic digest of β_h-EP. Lower, proposed primary structure of β_h-EP.

exceptions: (a) in steps 7 and 9, 5% *N*-methylmorpholine in CH_2Cl_2 (prepared fresh each day) was used; (b) steps 12 and 13 were deleted; (c) in step 16, 0.5 equivalent of *N*-methylmorpholine in TFE was used in place of the diisopropylethylamine (see Fig. 4). The last change has been found to be helpful in reducing nucleophilic attack on the *o*-BrZ protecting group of tyrosine when TFE is present, while, at the same time, it was effective in neutralizing the acid contamination in the Beckman 990-Peptide Synthesizer. The following side-chain protecting groups were employed: *o*-BrZ for Lys and Tyr; Bzl for Glu, Thr, and Ser. All amino acids, except glutamine and asparagine, were coupled by preforming the symmetrical anhydride of the Boc derivative in CH_2Cl_2 as described previously (Hagenmaier and Frank, 1972; Yamashiro and Li, 1974). The low solubility of Boc-Leu-OH in CH_2Cl_2 necessitated running this reaction with minimal cooling. Boc-Gln-OH was coupled by the symmetrical anhydride procedure in a DMF-CH_2-Cl_2 mixture (Hemmasi and Bayer, 1974), while Boc-Asn-OH was coupled by the DCC-1-hydroxybenzotriazole method (Konig and Geiger, 1970; Blake and Li, 1975). Since the beneficial effect of TFE in coupling efficiency is nullified by the presence of DMF, it was not used for coupling Boc-Gln-OH and Boc-Asn-OH. The Boc group of the last amino acid residue was removed with TFA. The yield of final protected peptide resin from 0.51 gm Boc(Bzl)Glu-bromo polymer (141 μmole) was 1.367 gm.

Protected β_h-EP bromo polymer (680 mg) was treated in HF (10 ml) for

Step	Operation and reagent	Mix time (min)
1	CH_2Cl_2, 12 ml (4 times)	1
2	55% Trifluoroacetic acid/CH_2Cl_2, 10 ml (once)	1
3	55% Trifluoroacetic acid/CH_2Cl_2, 7 ml (once)	15
4	CH_2Cl_2, 12 ml (3 times)	1
5	25% Dioxane/CH_2Cl_2, 12 ml (3 times)	1
6	CH_2Cl_2, 12 ml (3 times)	1
7	5% *N*-methylmorpholine/CH_2Cl_2, 12 ml (once)	2
8	CH_2Cl_2, 12 ml (2 times)	1
9	Repeat step 7	
10	Repeat step 8	
11	Repeat step 7	
12	CH_2Cl_2, 12 ml (6 times)	1
13	Symmetrical anhydride, 3 equivalents in 6.5 ml of CH_2Cl_2 (once)	20 and hold
14	0.5 Equivalent of *N*-methylmorpholine in TFE, 0.13 ml (once)	10
15	CH_2Cl_2, 12 ml (3 times)	1
16	33% Ethanol/CH_2Cl_2, 12 ml (3 times)	1

FIG. 4. Program for solid-phase synthesis of β_h-EP.

75 minutes at 0° in the presence of anisole (1.5 ml). After removal of HF, the oily residue was washed with ethyl acetate (25 ml). The product was extracted with 0.5 *N* acetic acid (5 ml) and subjected to gel filtration on a 2.16 × 25 cm column of Sephadex G-10 in 0.5 *N* acetic acid. A single peak was detected (280 nm), and isolation by lyophilization gave 272 mg. A portion (260 mg) upon gel filtration on a 2.5 × 137 cm column of Sephadex G-25 in 0.5 *N* acetic acid gave essentially one major peak, which on lyophilization gave 212 mg. A portion (206 mg) on CMC chromatography gave a major peak followed by a substantial second peak; isolation by lyophilization gave 119 and 48 mg, respectively. An aliquot of the major product (49 mg) was subjected to partition chromatography on Sephadex G-50 in a 1.76 × 47 cm column (Li *et al.*, 1976b) to give essentially one sharp symmetrical peak with R_f 0.37 (see Fig. 5), and isolation by lyophilization gave 33 mg (90% peptide content by amino acid analysis) of highly purified β_h-EP (32% yield based on starting resin). Figure 6 presents the synthetic scheme for β_h-EP.

Paper electrophoresis at pH 3.7 (pyridine acetate buffer) and pH 6.7 (collidine acetate buffer) for 4.5 hours at 400 V each gave a single spot (ninhydrin detection) with R_f values of 0.56 and 0.23 relative to lysine. Thin-layer chromatography in the solvent system of *n*-butanol–pyridine–HOAc–H_2O (5 : 5 : 1 : 4, v/v) gave one spot (ninhydrin) with R_f 0.52. A sample (12.4 mg) on partition chromatography in a 1.18 × 60 cm column of Sephadex G-50 gave the results in Fig. 5. Disc electrophoresis (0.1 mg) on a polyacrylamide gel at pH 4.5 gave one intense band. Amino acid analysis of a 24-hour HCl hydrolysis gave: $Lys_{5.3}Asp_{2.0}Thyr_{2.8}Ser_{1.7}Glu_{3.0}Pro_{1.0}Gly_{3.1}Ala_{1.8}Val_{1.0}Met_{0.9}Ile_{1.4}Leu_{2.1}Tyr_{1.9}Phe_{1.9}$ (the

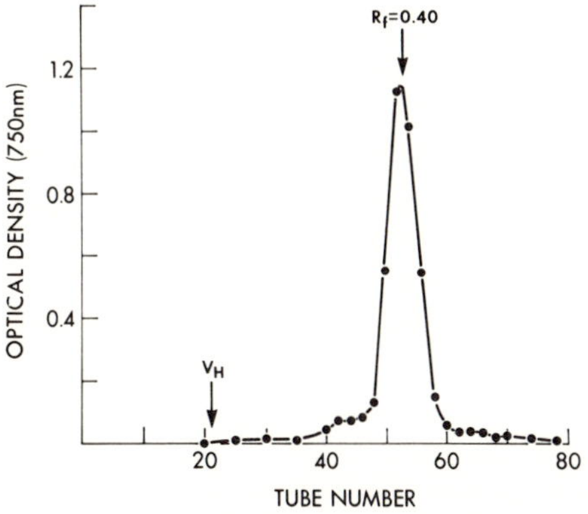

FIG. 5. Partition chromatography of synthetic β_h-EP (12.4 mg) on Sephadex G-50: column size, 1.18 × 60 cm; solvent system, 1-butanol-pyridine–0.6 *M* NH_4OAc (5 : 3 : 10); hold-up volume (V_h), 19 ml; 0.89 ml/tube; detection, Folin–Lowry method.

N^{α}-Boc-(Bzl)-Glu-Resin

1. TFA-CH_2Cl_2, 15 min
2. *N*-methylmorpholine
3. preformed symmetrical anhydride of Boc-Gly (CF_3CH_2OH to 20%)

↓

Boc-Gly-(Bzl)-Glu-Resin

1. TFA-CH_2Cl_2, 15 min
2. *N*-methylmorpholine
3. preformed symmetrical anhydride of Boc-AA (CF_3CH_2OH to 20%)

↓

Fully protected β_h-endorphin

1. TFA-CH_2Cl_2, 15 min
2. *N*-methylmorpholine

↓

Protected β_h-endorphin with free α-NH_2 group

1. HF, anisole, 0°, 75 min

↓

Crude β_h-endorphin

1. Sephadex G-10, 0.5 *N* HOAc
2. CMC chromatography
3. partition chromatography on G-50

↓

β_h-Endorphin (32% yield)

Resin, brominated styrene resin (1% divinylbenzene); side-chain protecting groups; Lys, Z(o-Br); His, Boc; Asp, Bzl; Thr, Bzl; Ser, Bzl; Glu, Bzl and Tyr (o-Br). Boc, tert-butyloxycarbonyl; Bzl, benzyl; TFA, trifluoroacetic acid; AA, amino acid.

FIG. 6. Synthetic scheme for β_h-EP.

Ile-Ile moiety is resistant). Amino acid analysis after complete enzymic digestion (first with trypsin and chymotrypsin and then leucine aminopeptidase) gave $Lys_{5.1}(Thr + Ser + Asn + Glu)_{7.7}Glu_{2.0}Pro_{1.1}Gly_{3.0}Ala_{1.8}Val_{1.1}Met_{1.0}Ile_{1.9}Leu_{2.1}Tyr_{2.0}Phe_{2.1}$.

For peptide mapping, a sample was treated in 0.23 ml of 0.2 *M* NH_4OAc, pH 8, with 26 μg trypsin at 37° for 6 hours. After repeated lyophilization, an aliquot was spotted in Whatman 3MM and mapped by chromatography in the solvent system of *n*-butanol–HOAc–H_2O (4 : 1 : 5, v/v) followed by electrophoresis (collidine acetate, pH 6.7, 400 V, 6 hours). Revelation by ninhydrin (0.01% in ethanol) gave five major spots (Fig. 7) that were cut out and extracted with 0.1 *N* NH_4OH for 24 hours. All minor spots were cut out and pooled for extraction. Amino acid analyses of HCl hydrolyzates gave for spot 1: $Lys_{1.0}Glu_{1.1}Gly_{0.9}$; spot 2, $Lys_{0.9}Thr_{1.1}Ser_{0.9}Glu_{1.2}Gly_{2.2}Met_{0.8}Tyr_{0.8}Phe_{1.1}$; spot 3, $Lys_{0.8}Thr_{1.9}Ser_{0.9}$

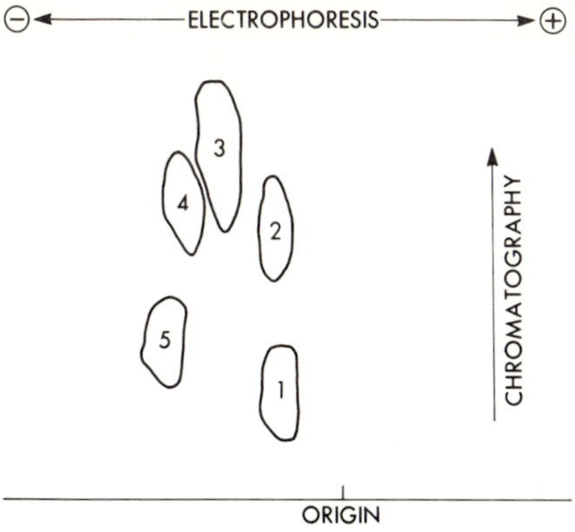

FIG. 7. Peptide map of tryptic digest of synthetic β_h-EP.

$Glu_{1.2}Pro_{0.9}Val_{1.0}Leu_{1.9}Phe_{1.1}$; spot 4, $Lys_{0.9}Asp_{1.0}Ala_{1.1}Ile_{1.7}$; spot 5, $Lys_{0.9}Asp_{1.1}Ala_{1.1}Tyr_{0.9}$. The five major spots accounted for 94% of the peptides detected by this procedure.

From the above data, it may be concluded that the synthetic β_h-EP is a homogeneous product.

V. Morphinelike Activity

The opiate activity of β_h-EP, as assayed by the guinea pig ileum preparation (Kosterlitz *et al.*, 1970) was comparable to that of the synthetic homolog and was blocked by the specific opiate antagonist naloxone (Table I). A somewhat lower potency for the natural product is most likely due to the fact that part of the methionine residue had been oxidized to sulfoxide during the isolation procedure. It may be noted in Table I that synthetic β_h-EP and β_c-EP had identical opiate activity. The amino acid sequence of β_c-EP (Li and Chung, 1976b) is identical to that of β_h-EP (Fig. 3) except that residues in positions 27 and 31 are His and Gln, respectively.

In the binding assay, β_c-EP was 3–5 times more potent than normorphine in competing for ^{3}H-opiate binding (Cox *et al.*, 1976). It elicited a positive Na^+ effect*, although the effect was comparatively smaller in

* The concentration of Na^+ in the medium of opiate-receptor assay proved to be the critical variable that differentiated agonist from antagonist binding (Snyder, 1975). The binding of agonists was found to be decreased by Na^+ whereas antagonist binding was increased.

TABLE I—Opiate Activity of β_h-Endorphin by Guinea Pig Ileum Assay

Preparation	IC_{50}[a] (*M*)	Relative potency: Normorphine	Relative potency: Syn. β_h-EP
Normorphine	2.50×10^{-7}	1.00	0.31
β_h-EP			
Synthetic	0.70×10^{-8}	3.58	1.00
Natural[b]	0.85×10^{-8}	2.94	0.82
β_c-EP, synthetic	0.70×10^{-8}	3.58	1.00

[a] IC_{50} was determined by plotting log molar concentration against mean percent inhibition. Normorphine and the peptides were assayed twice at four different concentrations. Dose-response curves of normorphine and the peptides were parallel.

[b] Natural β_h-endorphin at 1.2×10^{-7} *M* gave 58.5% inhibition and the inhibiting effect was completely reversed by naloxone (3.0×10^{-8} *M*).

magnitude than that of met-enkephalin (Bradbury *et al.,* 1976b). This might explain the weak *in vivo* activity of met-enkephalin and the potent analgesic response to β-EP (Loh *et al.,* 1976; Belluzi *et al.,* 1976). Interestingly, the parent molecule, β-LPH, and peptides with N-terminal sequence other than the pentapeptide, e.g., β-MSH (residues 41–58 of β-LPH), have no activity in the binding assay (Cox *et al.,* 1976; Bradbury *et al.,* 1976b).

For analgesic assays, male mice weighing 25–30 gm were used. The analgesic properties of β_h-EP were assessed in mice by the tail-flick method (D'Amour and Smith, 1941), the hot-plate method (Antier, 1974) and the acetic acid-induced writhing method (Koster *et al.,* 1959). The peptide was injected either intraventricularly (icv) in a volume of 5 μl according to the method described by Haley and McCormick (1957), or intravenously (iv) via the tail vein.

To evaluate the tail-flick and hot-plate responses, a control latency (T_0) was obtained from the mean of two latencies determined prior to drug injection; the test latencies (T_1) were determined at various times after injection for each animal. "Percent analgesia" was calculated as $[(T_1-T_0)/(T_2-T_0)] \times 100$, where the cut-off times (T_2) for the tail-flick and hot-plate tests were 10 and 60 seconds (Harris and Pierson, 1964), respectively. With a twofold increase in latency of reaction time of tail-flick response and hot-plate response as a quantal index of inhibition, the median analgesic dose (AD_{50}), and 95% confidence limits were calculated according to the method of Litchfield and Wilcoxon (1949). When "analgesia" was measured by the writhing method (Koster *et al.,* 1959), acetic acid (0.1 ml/10 gm body weight of 0.6% acetic acid) was administered intraperitoneally (ip) 5 minutes after the icv injection of β-EP. The number of writhing responses was counted for 10 minutes. To determine the AD_{50} for writhing, a quantal index of inhibited response was individually defined as any mouse that writhed less than twice after drug administration.

β_h-EP, at doses ranging from 0.09 to 0.38 μg per mouse injected icv, produced a dose-related inhibition of the tail-flick response of mice to this nociceptive heat stimulus (Fig. 8). This effect lasted 30–60 minutes, depending on the dose used. Subcutaneous injection of naloxone (1 mg/kg) 10 minutes after injection of β_h-EP completely reversed the analgesic response to the peptide. Similar results were obtained by the hot-plate test. Additionally, in the writhing assay, β_h-EP (0.38 μg per mouse injected 5 minutes before the injection of acetic acid) completely inhibited the writhing response to the stimulus of acetic acid. Pretreatment of mice with naloxone (HCl, 1 mg/kg sc) 5 minutes before the injection of β_h-EP completely abolished the inhibitory effect of β_h-EP on writhing.

In another experiment, β_h-EP was injected iv, and the analgesic response was again determined by the tail-flick method. β_h-EP, at doses of 9.4 mg/kg and 18.8 mg/kg, produced a dose-related inhibition of the tail-flick response after peripheral administration (Fig. 9). The effects lasted 20–30 minutes depending on the dose used. Pretreatment of mice with

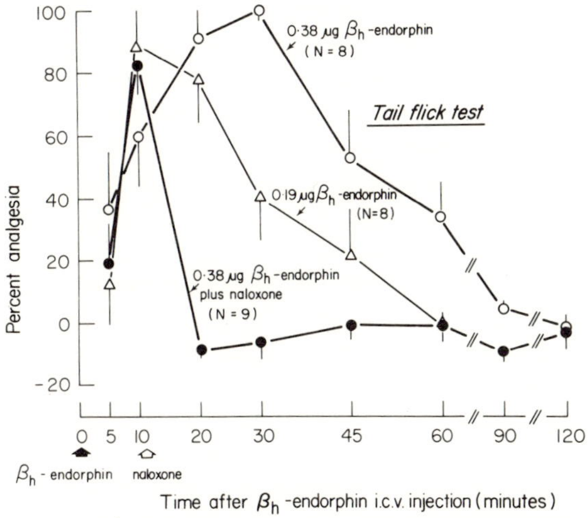

FIG. 8. Inhibitory effect on tail-flick response following icv injection of β_h-EP and its reversal by naloxone. β_h-EP was injected icv at 0 time (▲). Naloxone (1 mg/kg icv △) was injected at 10 minutes after β_h-EP. N, number of mice studies. The vertical bars indicate the SEM.

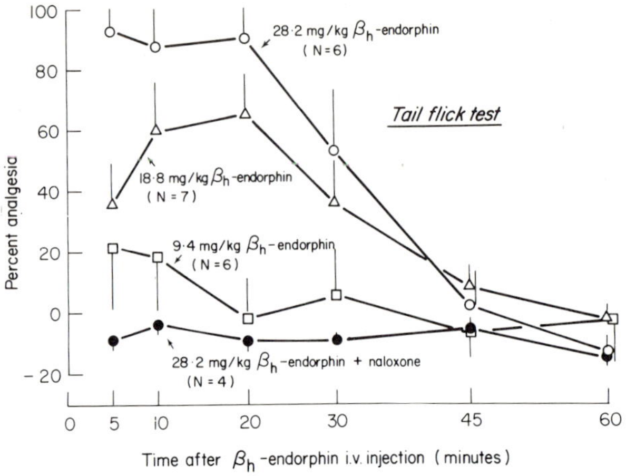

FIG. 9. Inhibitory effect on tail-flick response following iv injection of β_h-EP and its blockade by naloxone. β_h-EP was injected iv via the tail vein at 0 time. Naloxone HCl (1 mg/kg sc) was injected 5 minutes before the injection of β_h-EP. N, number of mice studies. The vertical bars indicate the SEM.

naloxone HCl (1 mg/kg sc) 5 minutes before the injection of 20.1 mg/kg of β_h-EP completely abolished the inhibitory effect of the peptide.

A quantitative determination of analgesic potency of β_h-EP after icv and iv injection is shown in Table II. Morphine is used as a reference compound for the comparison of potency with β_h-EP. When potency was compared on a molar basis, β_h-EP, when applied centrally, was 17–48 times more potent than morphine as estimated by the three bioassays. β_h-EP was 3.4 times more potent than morphine when injected iv (see Table II). Thus, the analgesic potency of β_h-EP is comparable to that of β_c-EP (Loh *et al.*, 1976).

VI. Development of Tolerance and Physical Dependence

It is widely recognized that opiates could easily develop tolerance and physical dependence. The concurrent development of these characteristics with chronic administration of morphine has led many investigators to believe that a common underlying or closely related mechanism operates within the matrix of the central nervous system. Chronic administration of opiates produces a dependent state that is generally characterized by abstinence behavior when opiate intake is abruptly terminated or when an opiate antagonist is administered.

In comparing the pharmacologic properties of opiatelike peptides to

TABLE II—Median Analgesic Doses (AD_{50}) of β_h-Endorphin in Mice

	AD_{50}[a] (nmole/mouse)	Potency ratio[a] (morphine = 1) Human	Camel
Intracerebroventricular injection			
Tail-flick test	0.026(0.017–0.043)	48.4	33.0
Hot-plate test	0.031(0.023–0.01)	32.8	17.5
Writhing test	0.026(0.017–0.40)	17.3	19.5
Intravenous injection			
Tail-flick test	3.32(1.86–5.69)[b]	3.4	3.5

[a] The values of AD_{50} of morphine and potency ratio for camel β-endorphin were obtained from our previous studies (Loh *et al.*, 1976). Values in parentheses are the 95% confidence limits of AD_{50}.

[b] μmole/kg.

opiate alkaloids, it is important to know if these peptides can produce tolerance and physical dependence. Met-enkephalin and β_c-EP were infused at two concentrations by the technique of Wei and Loh (1976). At the higher concentrations, naloxone precipitated in over 80% of the animals a withdrawal syndrome which was indistinguishable from that seen in morphine abstinent animals. The incidence of precipitated withdrawal was dose dependent, decreasing at lower doses of the peptides. Leu-enkephalin appeared to be devoid of dependence-producing properties.

As to the development of tolerance to repeated injections of the opiate peptide, β_h-EP was injected icv twice a day (at 9:00 A.M. and 4:30 P.M.) at a dose of 94 μg per rat. Rats showed analgesic effect to heat stimuli and catatonia for about 150–180 minutes after the first injection of 94 μg of peptide per rat. The durations of analgesic response and catatonia were gradually reduced after multiple injections of the same dose. On the fourth day, after six injections of 94 μg per rat of β_h-EP, rats showed only slight analgesic response and catatonia after injection of 37.6 μg per rat of the peptide; 18.8 μg per rat was shown to produce 100% analgesic response and strong catatonia for more than 1 hour in naive animals. Similar results were observed when 40 μg of morphine sulfate was injected.

VII. Cross-Tolerance to Morphine

Other characteristics of the pharmacologic effects of opiate alkaloids are cross-tolerance and cross-physical-dependence. In order to compare the pharmacologic effects of β-EP to opiates, as well as to elucidate the mechanism of β-EP actions, it is necessary to establish whether or not cross-tolerance and cross-physical-dependence exist between β-EP and morphine.

In these studies, rats were rendered tolerant to morphine by pellet-implantation techniquc as described by Way *et al.* (1969). The pellets were removed 72 hours after implantation. Five to six hours after pellet removal, rats were injected icv with 5 μl β_h-EP or morphine sulfate. The analgesic response of β_h-EP and morphine were assessed by the tail-flick method and the hot-plate method. On the other hand, the incidence of abrupt withdrawal jumping was used as an index for the quantitative measurement of physical dependence (Way *et al.*, 1969). In these studies, placebo-implanted rats injected with 1 μg of β_h-EP showed 80–100% analgesia in both the hot-plate and tail-flick tests. This effect lasted about 60 minutes. The same dose of β_h-EP produced much less inhibition in both the hot-plate and tail-flick responses to nociceptive stimuli in morphine-pellet-implanted rats.

A quantitative comparison of the analgesic potencies of β_h-EP and morphine in placebo-implanted and morphine-pellet-implanted rats is shown in Fig. 10. In placebo-pellet-implanted rats, the AD_{50} of β_h-EP was found to be 0.15 μg per rat in both the hot-plate and tail-flick tests, while the AD_{50} of morphine was 0.61 and 0.47 μg per rat, respectively, in these tests. When potency was compared on a molar basis, β_h-EP was 42 times

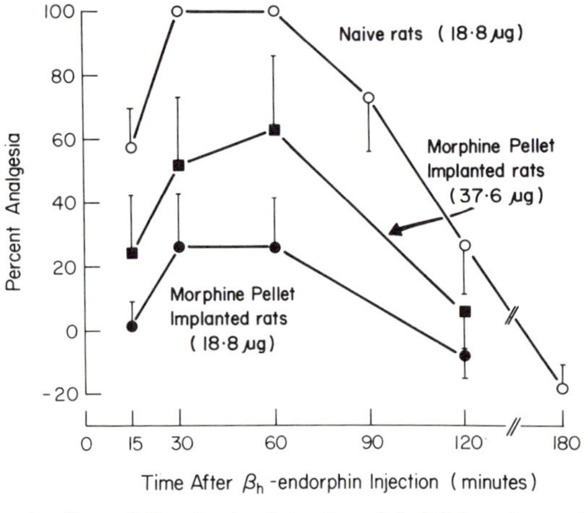

FIG. 10. Analgesic effects following icv injection of β_h-EP in naive and morphine-pellet-implanted rats, as measured by the tail-flick test. Rats, six per group, were rendered tolerant to morphine by implanting three morphine pellets, which were removed after 70 hours. Five hours after removal of the pellets, rats were injected with β_h-EP, 18.8 and 37.6 μg per rat at 0 time. The vertical bars indicate the SEM.

more potent than morphine in the hot-plate and 32 times more potent in the tail-flick test. The degree of cross-tolerance to β_h-EP was measured by the 8- to 9-fold increase of the AD_{50} of the peptide after morphine pellet implantation than that in placebo-implanted mice. A similar increase in the AD_{50} of morphine was found.

With regard to the suppression of withdrawal syndromes, in doses ranging from 0.043 to 0.17 μg per rat, β_h-EP caused a dose-related inhibition of abrupt withdrawal jumping in morphine-dependent rats. When the potency of the peptide was compared with that of morphine on a molar basis, β_h-EP was about 10 times more potent than morphine in the suppression of abrupt withdrawal jumping. Met-enkephalin, even in a high dose of 200 μg per mouse, did not suppress abrupt withdrawal jumping.

VIII. Experiments in the Cat

β_c-EP administered icv at doses of 25 and 50 μg in the cat (Meglio *et al.*, 1977) produced a dose-related inhibition of jaw-opening reflex (JOR) and response to nociceptive stimuli applied to the skin. This analgesic action of β_c-EP was accompanied by significant alteration in the animal's behavior. In fact, the behavioral alteration was observed at a dose of 12.5 μg without significant change in JOR or response to nociceptive stimuli. The analgesic effect and behavioral changes induced by the peptide lasted about 2 hours and resembled those induced by morphine sulfate, except that under morphine the cats were more excitable. These effects induced by β_c-EP at a dose of 25 μg were promptly and partially reversed by 0.8 mg/kg of naloxone administered ip.

A recovery period of at least 72 hours was allowed for each animal between drug administration and pharmacologic testing. This recovery period was essential because if β_c-EP was administered within less than 24 hours, there were observable alterations in the animal's behavior, but no analgesic effect of the peptide.

Hosobuchi *et al.* (1977) reported that β_c-EP developed tolerance and its reversal by 5-hydroxytryptophan (5-HTP). These investigators carried out experiments in eight cats that had stereotactically placed third ventricular cannulas (0.6 mm in shaft diameter) permanently fixed to the skull by means of acrylic resin. Synthetic β_c-EP was administered icv through this cannula in the awake, unrestrained cat. In all cats, the minimal effective dose (MED) of β_c-EP for analgesia by icv administration was 25 μg. Tolerance to the peptide developed acutely if administration was repeated within the first 24 hours. No analgesic effect was observed, although the behavioral alteration was present and lasted about 2 hours. This tolerance phenomenon was observed even if the initial dose of β_c-EP administered was below MED (12.5 μg) or when the second dose was above MED (50 μg). The analgesic effect of the peptide returned to original potency if the second administration was given after 48 hours. Throughout the testing, there was practically no change in the baseline threshold of JOR.

In four cats, 50 μg of β_c-EP was injected icv within 24 hours after the initial injection of 25 μg (MED); no analgesic effect was observed, although behavioral alterations occurred. After the second injection of the peptide, 1 hour was allowed to confirm that there was no delayed analgesic response (Fig. 11) to JOR. Within 10 minutes of ip administration of 5-HTP (10 mg/kg), a marked analgesic response was noted in JOR and peripheral pinch test in all four animals. The effect generally lasted 3–6 hours (Fig. 11).

A 3- to 4-fold increase in JOR and decreased or absent behavioral response to peripheral pinch was observed when 5-HTP was injected 40–60 minutes after icv administration of 12.5 μg (below MED) β_c-EP (Fig. 12). The analgesic effect was totally reversed by naloxone (ip 0.8 mg/kg). No augmentation of behavioral response associated with β_c-EP was observed.

The results of Hosobuchi *et al.* (1977) confirm previous observations (Meglio *et al.,* 1977) in the cat that a single administration of β_c-EP produces acute tolerance to its analgesic effect. Tolerance lasts at least 24 hours. During this period the animal seems also to develop cross-tolerance to morphine. Despite the development of acute tolerance to

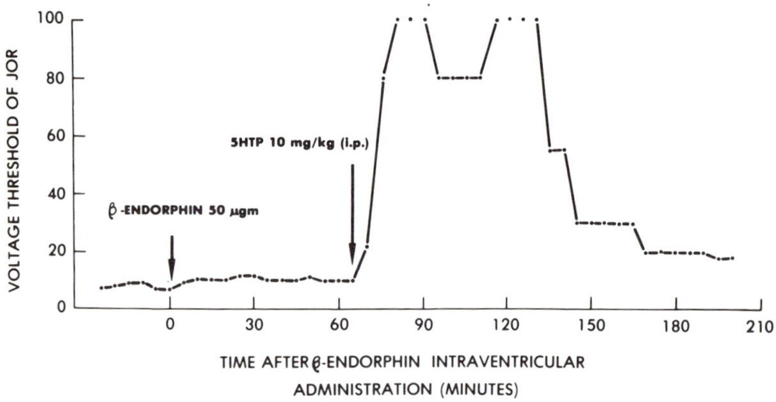

FIG. 11. The cat received icv 25 μg of β-EP 24 hours prior to 50 μg of the peptide administered icv. No alteration of JOR threshold was observed over 60 minutes. Ten to twenty minutes after the administration of 5-HTP ip produced marked analgesia in the animal, manifested by elevation of JOR threshold over 100 V and absence of behavioral response to peripherally applied noxious stimuli. This reversal effect lasted over 2 hours.

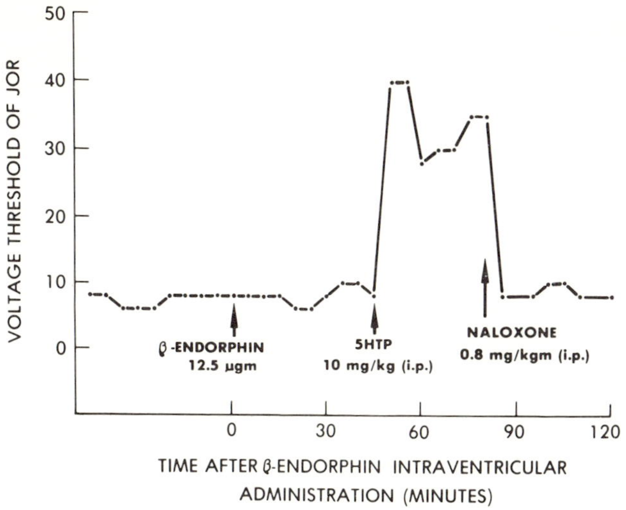

FIG. 12. No significant changes were observed in JOR threshold in this cat following icv administration of subliminal analgesic dose of β-EP (12.5 μg). 5-HTP produced an analgesic response, which was promptly blocked by ip naloxone, in the animals.

analgesic action, the behavioral effects elicited by β_c-EP persisted after injections for 3 days.

The acute tolerance induced by β_c-EP was reversed by systemic administration of 5-HTP, which is known to elevate the intracerebral serotonin content (Contreras *et al.*, 1973). 5-HTP also potentiated the analgesic effect of β_c-EP (Fig. 12). Contreras and co-workers reported a similar effect of 5-HTP in reducing tolerance development to morphine in mice (Tomayo and Contreras, 1965). Potentiation of the analgesic action of morphine by 5-HTP (Dewey *et al.*, 1970) has been reported, and similar findings were described by others (Saarnivaara, 1969; Way *et al.*, 1974). However, Way *et al.* found that 5-HTP accelerated the development of tolerance.

These data suggest that the analgesia produced by β_c-EP may be related to the activation of a serotonergic pathway. If the first dose of β_c-EP produced a reduction of serotonin in a given brain area, the second dose of the peptide might be expected to be noneffective. Its effects, however, could be restored by administration of the serotonin precursor, 5-HTP.

IX. Behavioral Activity in Rats

Other than the pharmacologic effects described above, Jacquet *et al.* (1976; Jacquet and Marks, 1976) described some behavioral effects of

β_c-EP and related peptides. Injections of met- and leu-enkephalins, as well as β_c-EP, directly into the brain resulted in a pronounced sedation and a state of immobility without motor paralysis. Reaching, tactile–placing, grasping, and biting reflexes, were depressed or abolished. The righting reflex disappeared when the subject was blindfolded. Following injection, animals became profoundly immobile (without muscular rigidity), maintaining unnatural postures without any attempt to return to a more normal position. This state of catatonia is reversible by naloxone, an opiate antagonist.

More recently, Bloom *et al.* (1976) also reported that β-EP produces a marked and prolonged state of catatonia; this effect occurs at molar doses 1/100–1/1000 times the analgesic threshold for the other opiatelike peptides or morphine.

When a dose of 94 μg of β_h-EP per rat was given icv, it caused profound hypothermia (Tseng *et al.*, 1977). The body temperature decreased at 30 minutes after injection and reached maximum hypothermia (4° lower than preinjection). Tolerance to the hypothermic effect of β_h-EP rapidly developed after multiple injections of β_h-EP, and no hypothermia was found at the third and fifth injection of β_h-EP (Fig. 13). Similar results were observed when 40 μg of morphine sulfate was injected.

β_h-EP at a dose of 18.8 μg per rat produced 100% analgesia and strong catatonia in naive rats. The same dose or double the dose of the peptide produced much less inhibition of tail-flick response to nociceptive stimuli and less catatonia in rats rendered tolerant to morphine pellet implantation for 3 days; 18.8 μg of β_h-EP caused hypothermia in naive animals. The body temperature decreased at 30 minutes after injection and reached maximum at 60 minutes (2.4° lower than preinjection), and hypothermia

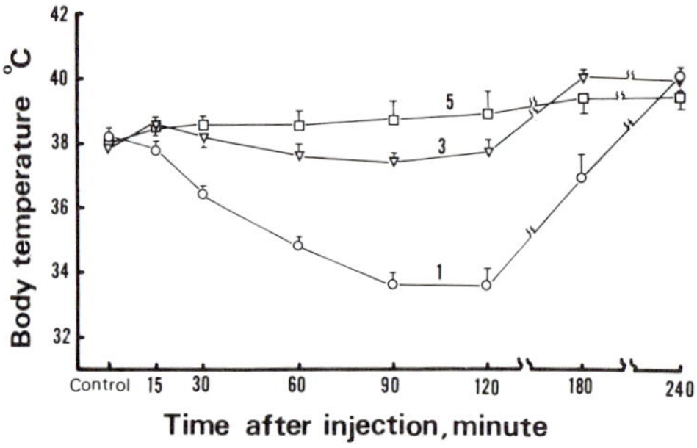

FIG. 13. Development of tolerance of hypothermic response to β_h-EP. Rats were injected icv with 94 μg of β_h-EP per rat twice a day for 3 days. On the fourth day, rats that were injected icv with 37.6 μg β_h-EP only caused slight inhibition of tail-flick response, whereas 18.8 μg of the peptide caused 100% inhibition of tail-flick response for 60–90 minutes in naive rats. The vertical bars indicate the SEM.

was produced at 120–240 minutes after injection. No hypothermia was found after injection of 18.8 and 37.6μg per rat of β_h-EP in morphine-pellet-implanted rats.

The salivation effect of β_c-EP was also observed (Holaday *et al.*, 1977). Injections of β_c-EP into the anterior horn of the lateral ventricle in rats produced a profound increase in salivation. This effect is most apparent with β_c-EP doses of 2–4 times the ED_{50} for analgesia, as measured by tail-flick latency, i.e., 10–20 μg in an injection volume of 20 μl. These doses of β_c-EP rendered the animals cataleptic; however, righting reflexes were usually maintained. In approximately 10–20% of animals receiving these doses of β_c-EP, copious salivation occurred, along with a behavioral pattern we describe as "sialogogic seizure." This is characterized by rhythmic opening of the mouth at about 1-second intervals, temporarily accompanied by movements of the forepaws that resemble an eating posture. Such sialogogic seizures were of 1 to 2-minute duration and generally occurred 3–4 times over a 20-minute interval. The onset of this behavior was 10–15 minutes after drug administration. If doses of β_c-EP are too excessive and righting reflexes lost, the animals may pass through the threshold for this seizure-like behavior to a state of complete catalepsy. The above describes sialogogic behavior as unique to β_c-EP, in that equivalent doses of morphine sulfate were never observed to produce salivation. A dose-response curve for this behavior based on a non-parametric rating has been obtained, and experiments are currently under way to evaluate naloxone reversibility, as well as possible biochemical mechanisms (Holaday *et al.*, 1977).

X. Structure–Activity Relationships

Table III lists the *in vitro* opiate activity of various peptides derived from β-EP. It is evident that β-EP is 3–10 times more potent than met-enkephalin. Omission of Gly-Glu at the COOH-terminus does not alter β-EP activity.

Opiate activities of the various peptides and enzymatic digests relative to β_c-EP as measured in the guinea pig ileum and rat brain receptor assays have been investigated by Doneen *et al*. (1977), and their results are summarized in Table IV. In the ileum assay, β_c-EP and β_h-EP were each 55% more potent than normorphine, and four-times more active than met-enkephalin. Similarly, in the opiate receptor assay, met-enkephalin had reduced potency (34%) compared to the β-EP's. β_h-LPH$^{61-69}$, corresponding to β_h-EP$^{1-9}$, was somewhat less potent than met-enkephalin. In contrast, β_s-LPH, β_h-LPH, and β_c-MSH showed no activity in either as-

TABLE III—Opiate Potency of Various Fragments of β-Endorphin

Residue no.	Assay procedure	Relative potency (normorphine = 1)
1–9	Guinea pig ileum[a]	0.4
1–5		0.9
1–31	Receptor binding[b]	5.3
1–5		0.2
1–31	Receptor binding[c]	1.6
1–29		1.6
1–5		0.5
1–31	Receptor binding[d]	0.1
1–16		0.002
1–9		0.01
1–5		0.02

[a] Gráf *et al.* (1976b).
[b] Cox *et al.* (1976).
[c] Bradbury *et al.* (1976b).
[d] Lazarus *et al.* (1976).

say, even when tested at the high concentration of 5.0×10^{-6}. β_s-LPH and β_c-MSH also failed to show naloxonelike antagonism to normorphine or β_c-EP in the ileum.

Acetone-treated β_h-EP, cyclized between Tyr[1]-Gly[2] by a bridge that incorporates the amino group of Tyr[1], displayed only 1% (ileum) and 2% (opiate receptor assay) of β_h-EP activity. β_h-EP, anisylated at its C-terminal glutamic acid residue, showed a modest decline in opiate activities. Whereas its amino-terminal Tyr may be essential, the carboxyl-terminal glutamic acid residue appears to contribute little directly to the interaction of β_h-EP with opiate receptors. In addition, conversion of Met[5] to 5-homoserine abolished the opiate activities of β_h-EP.

Hydrolysis of β_h-EP with chymotrypsin diminished considerably its potency in both assays. Chymotrypsin can be expected to cleave β_h-EP at Phe[4] as well as at other aromatic residues. On the other hand, digestion of β_h-EP with enzymes having no specificity within the amino-terminal five residues had no (carboxypeptidase A) or limited (trypsin) effects on *in vitro* opiate activities. Carboxypeptidase A has been shown to cleave the Gly[90]-Gln[91] dipeptide from porcine LPH[61–91] (Bradbury *et al.*, 1976b), indicating again the nonessential nature of these residues for opiate action. Trypsin digestion, however, reduced somewhat β_h-EP potency in ileum (71%) and opiate receptor binding (61%). Interestingly, these reduced activities were still greater than the activities of the nonapeptide β_h-

LPH^{61-69}, which can be expected to be produced by the action of trypsin on β_h-EP. Therefore, the trypsin digest contains either undigested β_h-EP or some other tryptic fragment, or fragments in combination, having opiate activity.

β_c-EP was susceptible to very limited hydrolysis with leucine aminopeptidase, as indicated by liberation of only trace amounts of tyrosine as detected by amino acid analysis. As shown in Table IV, this enzyme digest of β_c-EP showed only slight diminution of opiate activities; in contrast, met-enkephalin, which showed stoichiometric hydrolysis of the Tyr^1-Gly^2 bond, lost all activity after leucine aminopeptidase digestion. Therefore, the amino-terminal residue of β_c-EP appears to differ from that of met-enkephalin by being protected from exopeptidase attack. Enzymes in brain and plasma are known to rapidly inactivate enkephalins (Hambrook *et al.*, 1976), but digest less readily the more potent [D-Ala^2]-met-enkephalin (Pert *et al.*, 1976). The greater analgesic potency of β-EP compared to met-enkephalin *in vivo* may result, in part, from its greater resistance, especially at its amino terminus, to enzymic digestion.

TABLE IV—Opiate Activities of β_c-Endorphin and Related Peptides

Preparation	Relative potency[a] in: Guinea pig ileum	Relative potency[a] in: Brain opiate receptor binding
β_c-EP	1.00	1.00
β_h-EP	1.00	1.00
Met-enkephalin	0.25	0.34
Normorphine	0.65	—
β_s-LPH	<0.01	<0.01
β_h-LPH	<0.01	<0.01
β_c-MSH	<0.01	<0.01
β_h-$LPH^{(61-69)}$	0.20	0.26
Acetone-treated β_h-EP	0.01	0.02
(Antisylated-Glu^{31})-β_h-EP	0.76	0.75
Formic acid-treated-β_h-EP	1.00	1.00
(5-Homoserine)-β_h-EP	<0.01	<0.01
β_h-EP:carboxypeptidase A digest	1.00	1.00
β_h-EP:chymotryptic digest	0.13	0.03
β_h-EP:tryptic digest	0.71	0.61
β_c-EP:leucine aminopeptidase digest	0.97	0.93
Met-enkephalin:leucine aminopeptidase digest	<0.01	<0.01

[a] Potency of β_c-EP is defined as 1.00. Other preparations were compared to β_c-EP standard on a molar basis. IC_{50} of β_c-EP: 2.5–8.0 × 10^{-8} *M* in the guinea pig ileum assay; 1.2–3.7 × 10^{-7} *M* in the rat brain opiate receptor-binding assay.

XI. Synthesis and Biologic Activity of β-Endorphin Analogs with D-Amino Acids in Residue Positions 1, 2, 4, and 5

In order to examine the stereochemical requirements for morphinelike activity in the enkephalin segment of β-EP, the following analogs have been synthesized (Yamashiro *et al.*, 1977) by the solid-phase method using the same tactics as for the synthesis of β_c- and β_h-EP (Li *et al.*, 1976a; Li *et al.*, 1977a): [D-Tyr[1]]-, [D-Ala[2]]-, [D-Phe[4]]-, and [D-Met[5]]-β_c-EP. Purification of these synthetic peptides was effected by gel filtration on Sephadex G-10, chromatography on CMcellulose, and partition chromatography on Sephadex G-50. Three of the four analogs proved to be readily separable from β_c-EP by partition chromatography on Sephadex G-50 in the solvent system 1-butanol–pyridine–0.6 *M* NH_4OAc (5 : 3 : 10 *v/v;* pH of lower phase, 8.2). Overall yields based on starting Boc-Gln-Bromopolymer and on peptide content by amino acid analysis: [D-Tyr[1]]-β_c-EP, 20%; [D-Ala[2]]-β_c-EP, 25%; [D-Phe[5]]-β_c-EP, 27%; and [D-Met[5]]-β_c-EP, 35%.

Tables V and VI present the *in vitro* and *in vivo* assay data for opiate activity of these four synthetic analogs. The [D-Ala[2]]-β_c-EP possessed 100% analgesic potency compared with that of the parent molecule in *in vivo* assays (Table VI). There seems to be little correlation between these two assay systems in opioid peptides. It appears that *in vitro* assay in guinea pig ileum is not a reliable test to predict the *in vivo* analgesic activity for morphinelike peptides. The fact that [D-Ala[2]]-β_c-EP has the same potency as the parent molecule is in sharp contrast to the greater analgesic activity (Pert *et al.*, 1976) of [D-Ala[2]]-enkephalinamide over that of met-enkephalin.

The other three analogs exhibit drastic decreases in biologic activity (Tables V and VI), which indicates the importance of the stereochemical relationships of the side-chain functions to each other in the enkephalin segment. However, it may be noted that [D-Met[5]]-β_c-EP still possesses

TABLE V—Opiate Activity of Synthetic β_h-Endorphin Analogs by Guinea Pig Ileum Assay

Preparations	IC_{50} (*M*)	Relative potency[a]
β_c-Endorphin	2.7×10^{-8}	100
[D-Tyr[1]]-β_c-EP	2.9×10^{-6}	≤1
[D-Ala[2]]-β_c-EP	6.3×10^{-8}	43
[D-Phe[4]]-β_c-EP	6.7×10^{-7}	4
[D-Met[5]]-β_c-EP	6.6×10^{-7}	4

[a] Relative potencies are calculated using the IC_{50} of β_c-endorphin as 100%.

TABLE VI—Analgesic Potency of Synthetic β_c-Endorphin and Analogs in Mice

Preparation	AD_{50}[a]	Relative potency[b]
Morphine sulfate	0.42 (0.36–0.49)	2.9
β_c-endorphin	0.11 (0.07–0.17)	100.0
[D-Tyr[1]]-β_c-EP	22.5 (13.4–37.8)	0.5
[D-Ala[2]]-β_c-EP	0.11 (0.08–0.17)	100.0
[D-Phe[4]]-β_c-EP	>43	<0.3
[D-Met[5]]-β_c-EP	11.48 (7.17–18.36)	1.0

[a] AD_{50} in μg/25 g mouse (95% confidence limit).
[b] The relative potencies are calculated on molar basis using the AD_{50} of β_c-endorphin as 100%.

analgesic activity (Table VI) inasmuch as β_c-EP is much more active than morphine in these assays.

XII. Synthesis and Biologic Activity of β-Endorphin Analogs with Shortened Peptide Chains

As noted in Section X, the "nonenkephalin" segment (residues 6–31) plays an important role in the unique actions of β-EP, but it is not clear whether this entire segment is necessary for these actions. In order to explore the contribution of the nonenkephalin segment of β-EP to its biologic behavior, β_c-EP-(1–5)-(28–31), β_c-EP-(6–31), and β_h-EP-(1–5)-(16–31) were synthesized by the solid-phase method and their biologic properties investigated (Li *et al.*, 1977c).

As summarized in Table VII, only β_c-EP-(1–5)-(16–31) was found to

TABLE VII—Morphinelike Activity of Synthetic β-Endorphin Analogs

		In vivo analgesic activity	
Synthetic peptides	*In vitro* opiate activity[a]	AD_{50}[b]	Relative potency[c]
β_c-EP	100	0.11 (0.07–0.17)	100
β_c-EP-(6–31)	4	>86	<0.1
β_h-EP-(1–5)-(16–31)	135	25.1 (16.8–37.1)	0.3
β_c-EP-(1–5)-(28–31)	35	>86	<0.1

[a] Taken from Li *et al.*, 1977b.
[b] AD_{50} in μg/mouse (95% confidence limit); 7–10 mice for each dose tested.
[c] Molar basis.

exhibit significant analgesic activity with relative potency to the parent peptide of 0.3% and the analgesia was only partially, not completely, blocked by naloxone. In addition to the inhibition of the tail-flick response, mice became extremely hyperactive to sound and touch, attempting to jump out of their cages and escape. The analgesic response and hyperactivity lasted 10 to 20 minutes. However, the hyperactive response was not antagonized by pretreatment with naloxone (3 mg/kg), indicating that the response is not mediated via opiate like mechanisms.

β_c-EP-(1–5)-(28–31) was not active at a dose of 42.5 μg. β_c-EP-(6–31) at doses of 42.5 and 85 μg produced analgesia in one out of five and four out of eleven mice, respectively; the inhibition of the tail flick response by this peptide in some mice did not appear to be an opioid action. It is important to note that β_c-EP-(6–31) does not contain the enkephalin segment and yet it appears to possess measurable analgesic activity. However, it is evident that the entire amino acid sequence of β-EP is necessary for full analgesic activity *in vivo*.

XIII. Extraanalgesic Activity

Loh, Way, and their co-workers (Brase and Sampath-Khanna, 1976; Sampath-Khanna *et al.*, 1977) have shown that potassium-induced ^{3}H-labeled dopamine release from superfused striatal tissue from several strains of mice that exhibit running activity in response to morphine can be inhibited by 10^{-5} M morphine. This inhibition of dopamine release appears to be a specific opiate effect because it is antagonized by naloxone and because striatal tissue from mice made tolerant to morphine by morphine pellet implantation for 3 days exhibits tolerance to the inhibitory effect of morphine on dopamine release *in vitro* (Sampath-Khanna *et al.*, 1977).

In Table VIII, the effects of morphine, β_c-EP and met-enkephalin on the net tritium overflow induced by the depolarizing concentration of potassium chloride are compared. β_c-EP was about twice as potent as morphine; the IC_{50} for β_c-EP was 1.0 μM and that of IC_{50} for morphine was 2.2 μM. Met-enkephalin, on the other hand, did not produce a significant inhibition of tritium overflow in concentrations as high as 100 μM. Naloxone, at an equimolar concentration, produced a significant blockade of the inhibition by morphine and β-EP, the blockade being more complete in the presence of the peptide.

This is the first demonstration of an inhibition of neurotransmitter release from central nervous system tissue by an endogenous opiatelike

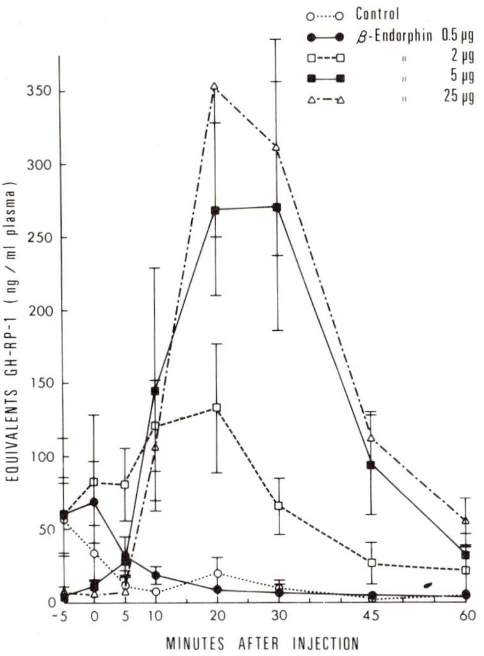

FIG. 14. Effect of increasing doses of β-EP on plasma GH levels in the rat. Male rats bearing intraventricular and intrajugular cannulae were injected iv with 0.2 ml of sheep somatostatin antiserum 5 minutes before the icv injection of the indicated amounts of synthetic β-EP. GH measurements were performed at the indicated time intervals after administration of β-EP. Data are presented as mean ± SEM.

peptide. The actions of β_c-EP in the central nervous system are probably not limited to the inhibition of dopamine release, as it is known that opiate drugs also inhibit the release of acetylcholine (Beleslin and Polak, 1965; Howes *et al.*, 1970; Matthews *et al.*, 1973; Waterfield *et al.*, 1976) and norepinephrine (Montel *et al.*, 1974; Jhamandas *et al.*, 1975) from CNS tissue. At the present time, however, dopamine is the only neurotransmitter for which tolerance to the effect of morphine *in vitro* has been demonstrated with CNS tissue and for which an inhibition of real release by morphine has been correlated, at least qualitatively, with a behavioral effect of morphine by utilizing mouse strain differences (Brase and Sampath-Khanna, 1976; Sampath-Khanna *et al.*, 1977).

Morphine is known to be a potent stimulant of somatotropin release in the rat (Kokka *et al.*, 1972; Ferland *et al.*, 1976a,b). This opiate effect is likely to be mediated by increased release of somatotropin-releasing fac-

TABLE VIII—Opiate Inhibition of Striatal Tritium Overflow and Reversal by Naloxone

Drug	Concentration (M)	Net overflow (%)
Morphine	0	17.69 ± 2.69 (13)
Morphine	1.0×10^{-6}	16.14 ± 3.42 (8)
Morphine	3.0×10^{-6}	5.04 ± 1.17[a] (10)
Morphine	1.0×10^{-5}	0.41 ± 0.25[a] (5)
Morphine + naloxone	3.0×10^{-6}	16.85 ± 3.02 (8)
β-Endorphin	0	20.04 ± 2.99 (4)
β-Endorphin	0.6×10^{-6}	16.76 ± 3.62 (4)
β-Endorphin	1.2×10^{-6}	8.06 ± 1.60[a] (4)
β-Endorphin	3.0×10^{-6}	0.12 ± 0.12[a] (4)
β-Endorphin + naloxone	3.0×10^{-6}	10.70 ± 2.72[b] (4)
Enkephalin	0	18.09 ± 2.44 (7)
Enkephalin	1.0×10^{-5}	20.99 ± 4.70 (8)
Enkephalin	1.0×10^{-4}	17.23 ± 4.11 (5)

[a] Significantly different from control ($p = 0.02$ or less).

[b] Significantly different from 3×10^{-6} M β-endorphin alone ($p < 0.01$).

Net overflow was calculated from tritium in fractions 11–15 corrected for the estimated spontaneous tritium overflow and is expressed as a percentage (mean ± SEM) of the total tritium in the striatal slice at the beginning of the collection of fraction 11. Numbers in parentheses indicate the number of experiments.

tor from the hypothalamus (Ferland *et al.*, 1977). In a study to determine the effect of β-EP and its related peptides on somatotropin release, it was found (Dupont *et al.*, 1977a) that 2 μg of β-EP injected icv in rats pretreated with antisomatostatin serum led to a 6- and 10-fold stimulation of the plasma somatotropin concentration measured 10 and 20 minutes after injection of the peptide, whereas 400 μg met-enkephalin led to a 4- to 6-fold increase in plasma somatotropin levels at 10 minutes, with a rapid return to basal levels at later time intervals. At doses of 5 and 25 μg, β-EP led to a 20- and 30-fold stimulation of plasma somatotropin levels, the maximal effect being measured between 20 and 30 minutes after injection (Fig. 14). These data suggest the possible role of the endogenous opiatelike peptides in the control of somatotropin.

Morphine is also known to stimulate the release of prolactin (Meites, 1966; Tilis *et al.*, 1975). It is not surprising that β-EP exhibits prolactin-release* in the rat by icv injection (Dupont *et al.*, 1977b).

* Similar studies on the *in vivo* effect of β-EP on somatotropin and prolactin release were reported by Rivier *et al.* (1977).

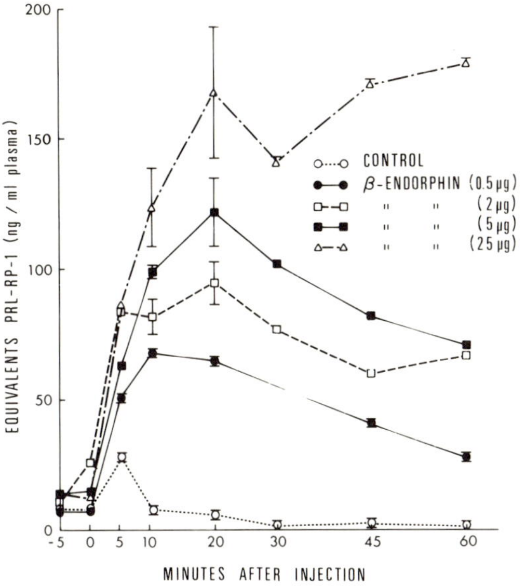

FIG. 15. Effect of increasing doses of β-EP on plasma prolactin (PRL) levels in the rat. Adult male rats bearing intraventricular and intrajugular cannulae were injected iv with 0.2 ml of sheep somatostatin antiserum 5 minutes before the icv injection of the indicated amounts of synthetic β-EP. PRL measurements were performed at the indicated time intervals after administration of β-EP. Data are presented as mean ± SEM of triplicate measurements of pooled plasma samples from eight to nine animals per group.

As illustrated in Fig. 15, the icv injection of 0.5–25 μg of β-EP led to a rapid and significant stimulation of PRL release in unanesthetized freely moving rats. With the 0.5 μg dose, a marked rise was already evident 5 minutes after injection of the peptide, and a maximal stimulation (approximately sevenfold) was measured after 10 minutes, with a slow decrease of plasma hormone levels at later time intervals. The higher doses of β-EP (2.5 and 25 μg) led to a progressive increase of PRL release, a 30- to 60-fold increase being measured between 20 and 60 minutes after injection of 25 μg of the peptide.

Many hormones have been shown to alter gene expression, resulting in stimulation of both protein and/or RNA synthesis in target cells and, in some instances, inhibition of protein synthesis (Hamilton, 1968; Tata, 1970). β-EP causes an increase in template activity of calf thymus DNA (Lee *et al.*, 1977). The stimulation is concentration related (Table IX) and sensitive to rifampicin, since the drug at 0.03 μg/ml would abolish completely the stimulatory effect induced by β-EP. Stimulation of template activity by the peptide requires the presence of both the primer and RNA polymerase.

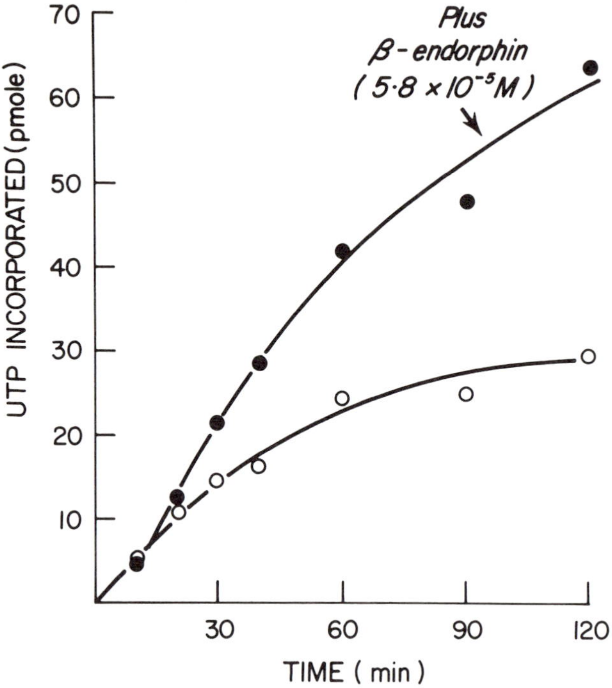

FIG. 16. Effect of β-EP on DNA-dependent ^{3}H-labeled UTP incorporation. Five units of *Escherichia coli* K-12 RNA polymerase and calf thymus DNA, 0.02 μg, were incubated in 0.25 ml, at 37° for 60 minutes. Reaction mixture contains Tris–HCl, 80 m*M* (pH 8.3, 23°), 100 m*M* NaCl, 4 m*M* $MgCl_2$, 2 m*M* $MnCl_2$, 6 m*M* dithiothreitol, 20 μg bentonite, 1 m*M* each of GTP, ATP, and CTP and 0.25 m*M* ^{3}H-labeled UTP ($2–3 \times 10^6$ cpm) and with or without 5.8×10^{-5} *M* β-EP. The reaction was stopped by the addition of 1 ml of 10% trichloroacetic acid containing 5% sodium pyrophosphate and 150 μg bovine serum albumin. After 15 minutes at 0°, the precipitates were filtered on glass fiber filters (Whatman GF/C) and washed 4 times with 9 ml 5% TCA + 3% PP_i and once with 9 ml cold ethanol. The filters were dried and counted in 9 ml Scientiverse in Beckman LS-100 scintillation counter.

TABLE IX—Template Activity of β-Endorphin

Peptide	Conc. ($10^{-5}M$)	Specific activity (^{3}H-UTP incorporation, nmoles/mg DNA)	Stimulation (%)
No addition	0	1.02	0
β-Endorphin	3	1.89	85
	6	2.30	125

Figure 16 shows the time course of ^{3}H-labeled UTP incorporation with or without 5.8×10^{-5} *M* β-EP. Without the peptide, ^{3}H-labeled UTP incorporation is linear up to 60 minutes and reaches a plateau. With β-EP, there is no apparent effect before 20 minutes; however, incorporation is then stimulated and continues up to 120 minutes. β-EP also stimulates ^{3}H-labeled UTP incorporation when the DNA primer is mouse brain chromatin (Fig. 17). The response is linear with the amount of chromatin present. In all studies reported, β-EP fulfilled the requirements needed to be considered as an endogenous opiate. However, Lee *et al*. (1977) found that morphine sulfate, up to 10^{-4} *M*, has no effect on template activity *in vitro*. Furthermore, the stimulation induced by β-EP is not reversed by $10^{-4}M$ of naloxone.

XIV. Radioimmunoassay: Dissociation of Opiate Activity and Immunoreactivity

A sensitive radioimmunoassay for β_h-EP has been developed (Li *et al*., 1977b). Rabbits were immunized with β_h-EP and guinea pigs with the

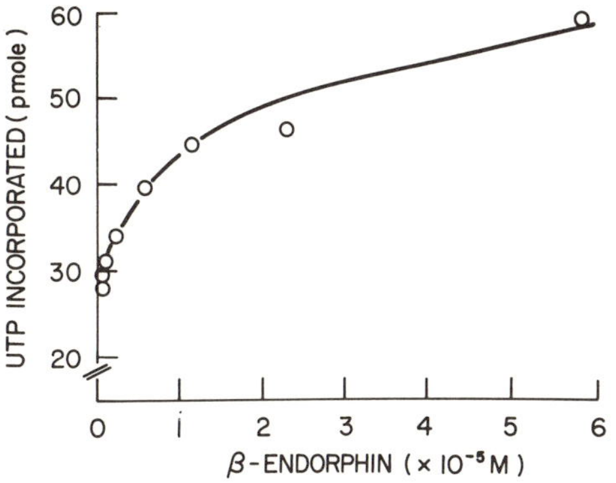

FIG. 17. Effect of β-EP on brain chromatin dependent ^{3}H-UTP incorporation assay procedure is the same as described in Fig. 16.

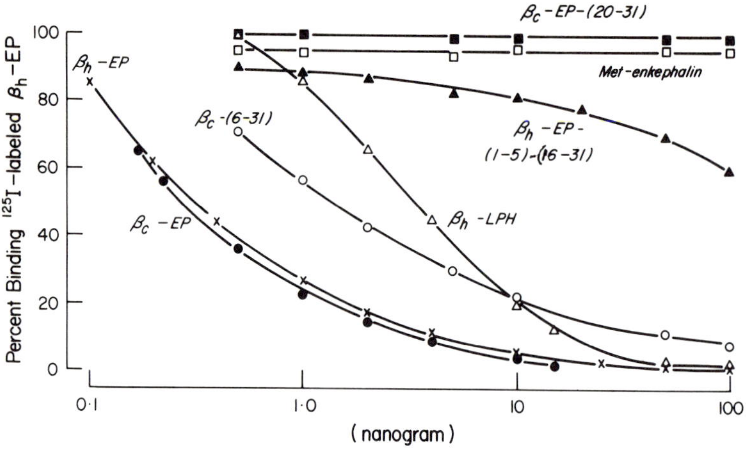

FIG. 18. Competition of β_c-EP, β_c-EP^{6-31}, β_h-LPH, β_h-EP, β_h-$EP^{(1-5)+(16-31)}$, β_c-EP^{20-31} and met-enkephalin in the β_h-EP RIA. Final dilution of antiserum was 1 : 3000.

EP-γ-globulin conjugate. The serum was checked for the presence of antibodies by testing its ability to bind ^{125}I-labeled β_h-EP, which was prepared by the lactoperoxidase method. The specific activity of the iodinated hormone was 85 mCi/mg. Separation of the free iodine and iodinated hormone was done by chromatography on Sephadex G-25 equilibrated with 0.1 *N* acetic acid.

For RIA, approximately 7000–8000 cpm of [^{125}I]-β_h-EP in 0.1 ml, various quantities of unlabeled β_h-EP, or other related peptides in 0.1 ml were incubated with 0.1 ml of antiserum to β_h-EP in the cold at 4° for a period of 16–20 hours. All dilutions for RIA were carried out in 0.01 *M* sodium phosphate buffer, pH 7.5, containing 0.15 *M* NaCl, 1% bovine serum albumin, and 0.33% EDTA in 12 × 75 mm glass tubes. Separation of the bound and free hormone was achieved by addition of 0.5 ml of phosphate buffer, pH 7.5, containing 20 mg Norit and 10 mg dextran T-70 (Pharmacia, Uppsala) per milliliter. The tubes were allowed to stand in cold for 10 minutes after which they were centrifuged for 30 minutes in the cold at 5000 rpm. The clear supernatant (0.5 ml) was mixed with 5 ml of scintillation fluid (PCS) and counted in a Packard β-counter. The procedure for counting γ-radiation in β-counter was essentially that of Herscowitz and McKillip (1974).

As shown in Fig. 18, the sensitivity of RIA for β_h-EP was in the range of 0.1–1.4 ng. β_c-EP gave a completely parallel and almost identical inhibition curve. β_c-EP^{6-31} also exhibited a parallel inhibition curve but had 40% immunoreactivity, as compared with β_c-EP. On the other hand, β_c-$EP^{(1-5)+(16-31)}$ showed very weak cross-reaction. It may be noted that β_h-

LPH, which contains the complete amino acid sequence of β_h-EP, had only 10% immunoreactivity. Figure 18 also shows that β_c-EP$^{20-31}$ and met-enkephalin, (β_c-EP$^{1-5}$) did not show any cross-reactivity. Thus, it is probable that β_c-EP$^{6-15}$ represents the antigenic determinant of β-EP.

Figure 19 presents logarithmic dose-response curves in the ileum preparation. It is evident that β_c-EP$^{(1-5)+(16-31)}$ is more active than the parent molecule, yet it shows very weak immunoreactivity by RIA (see Fig. 18). Met-enkephalin possesses significant *in vitro* opiate activity but shows no immunoreactivity. β_c-EP$^{6-31}$ is immunoreactive, but it has minimal opiate activity. Interestingly, β_h-LPH is immunoreactive, but it has very low opiate activity. These data clearly show that there is no correlation between opiate activity and immunoreactivity.

XV. Concluding Remarks

Biologically active compounds are generally isolated on the basis of certain biologic effects that have been observed by experimental scientists

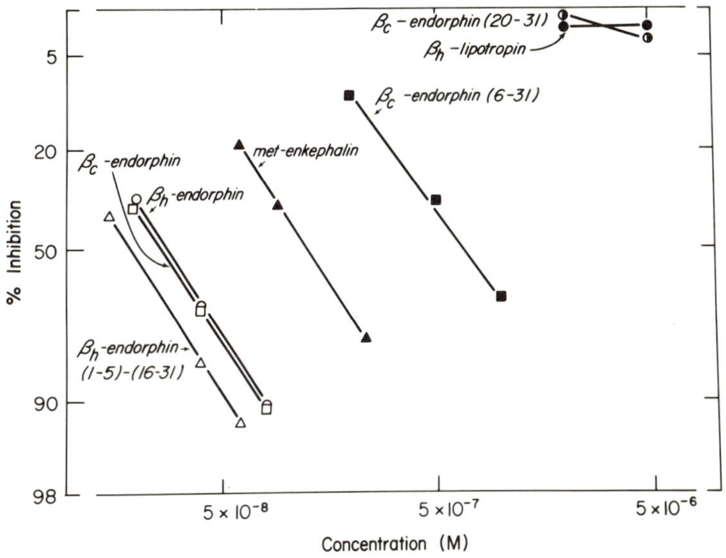

FIG. 19. Guinea pig ileum bioassay of β-EP and its fragments. IC_{50} (50% inhibiting concentration) of β_h-EP was 2.71 and 2.69×10^{-8} *M*, respectively. The relative potencies of the peptides were as follows: β_h-EP and β_c-EP, 1.00; met-enkephalin, 0.26; β_c-EP-(6–31), 0.04; β_h-EP$^{(1-5)+(16-31)}$, 1.35; β_c-EP$^{30-31}$, ≤ 0.001; β_h-LPH, ≤ 0.001. The inhibition of ileum concentration by β_c-EP$^{6-31}$ appears not to act through the opiate receptor as its effect was of unusually short duration (<12 seconds) and was not blocked by the specific opiate antagonist, naloxone.

or clinicians. The development of endocrinology has depended chiefly upon these observations. Many early discoveries of hormonal principles were derived from the removal of endocrine glands and the subsequent observations of the effect of this removal on the whole organism. Later chemists or biochemists investigated extracts of that particular gland, isolated the active substance in pure form, determined its structure, and synthesized the product in the laboratory.

This has been the classical way in which biomedical science has progressed. Certainly, it was this approach that gave the first clues concerning the existence of the hormonal principles which are known to us at present, and had it not been used, there undoubtedly would have been great delays in obtaining therapeutically useful compounds in medicine.

Another approach, one that has not been given much attention in the past, is coming to take its place alongside the biologic approach. This involves isolating a chemical compound from its natural source and investigating its biologic activity after it has been determined to be a pure substance.

An example is the discovery of β-LPH in 1964 (Li, 1964). This originated from a purely chemical investigation. In the course of improving the method for the isolation of ACTH from sheep glands (Birk and Li, 1964), we obtained a new peptide that differs completely from all other known pituitary hormones. Its biologic behavior was tested after it had been characterized chemically. Although the complete amino acid sequence of β-LPH was determined by Li *et al.* in 1965, some investigators still questioned whether it was a hormone or a new biologically active peptide from the anterior lobes of pituitary glands.

The discovery of β-EP was also achieved by the chemical approach. In the early 1970's, we had been investigating various hormones from camel pituitaries (Li *et al.,* 1975). When camel pituitary extract was submitted to fractionation on ion-exchange resin chromatography in the same manner as for the isolation of sheep β-LPH, we were not able to find camel β-LPH, but we did isolate a 31-amino acid peptide with very little lipolytic activity. This was achieved in January 1974. Subsequently, the primary structure of the 31-amino acid peptide was established in November 1974, to be the sequence (residues 61–91) of the COOH-terminal 31-amino acids in the sheep β-LPH molecule (Li *et al.,* 1965, 1966; Li and Chung, 1976b). After it was assayed for the *in vitro* opiate activity in December 1975, it was designated β-endorphin (β-EP) (Li and Chung, 1976a).

In Fig. 20, the amino acid sequence of bovine (Geschwind *et al.,* 1957) and human (Harris, 1959; Pickering and Li, 1963) β-melanotropins occupy residues 41–58 and 37–58 in the structure of ovine β-LPH, respectively. γ-Lipotropin (Chrétien and Li, 1967) is the NH_2-terminal 58-residue frag-

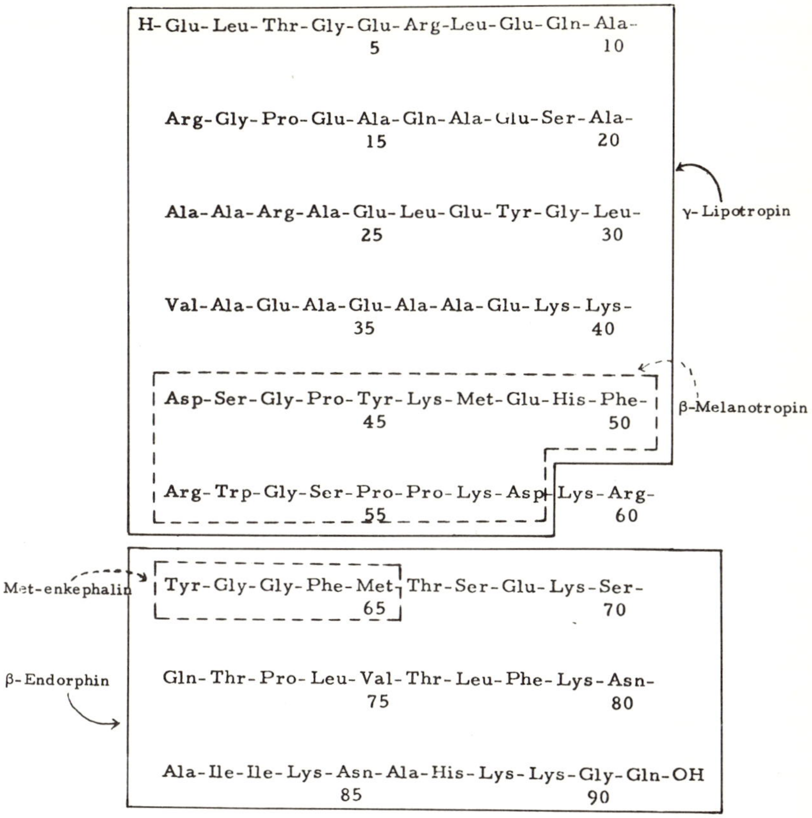

FIG. 20. Structural relationship of γ-lipotropin, β-melanotropin, met-enkephalin, and β-EP to ovine β-lipotropin.

ment in β-LPH. Besides met-enkephalin (residues 61–65) and β-EP (residues 61–91), β-LPH$^{61-69}$, β-LPH$^{61-76}$, β-LPH$^{61-77}$, and β-LPH$^{61-79}$ possess *in vitro* opiate activity (Gráf *et al.*, 1976b,c; Li and Chung, 1976a; Ling *et al.*, 1976; Doneen *et al.*, 1977). It has been proposed by various investigators (Chrétien and Li, 1967; Chrétien *et al.*, 1976a; Cox *et al.*, 1976; Lazarus *et al.*, 1976) that β-LPH serves as a prohormone for the biologically active peptides. Indeed, Gráf and Kenessey (1976) showed that incubation of β-LPH with pituitary homogenate causes the cleavage of a single peptide bond Leu-Phe at sequence positions 77–78 of the hormone.

Among various fragments of β-LPH having opiate activity, only β-EP exhibits potent analgesic activity by iv injections. In addition, it is the most active fragment when administered directly into the brain. Investigations of its structure–activity relationships will provide a clue to the development of a peptide with antagonistic action to alkaloid narcotics. It may also lead to the development of a peptide with potent analgesic activity, but no addictive property. As has been speculated by some investigators (Jacquet and Marks, 1976; Bloom *et al.,* 1976), β-EP and its related peptides may be linked to schizophrenia and other forms of mental diseases.

Acknowledgement

I thank the following colleagues for their contributions in these investigations on β-endorphin: D. Chung, D. Yamashiro, B. A. Doneen, A. J. Rao, H. H. Loh, L. F. Tseng, and Y. Hosobuchi. This work was supported in part by the National Institutes of Health and the Allen-Geffen Fund.

References

Antier, S. (1974). *Eur. J. Pharmacol.* **27,** 1–4.
Beckett, A. H. (1959). *Fortschr. Arzneimittelforsch* **1,** 455–530.
Beleslin, D., and Polak, R. L. (1965). *J. Physiol. (London)* **177,** 411–419.
Belluzzi, J. D., Grant, N., Garsky, V., Sarantakis, D., Wise, C. D., and Stein, L. (1976). *Nature (London)* **260,** 625–626.
Birk, Y., and Li, C. H. (1964). *J. Biol. Chem.* **239,** 1048–1052.
Blake, J., and Li, C. H. (1975). *Int. J. Pep. Protein Res.* **7,** 495–501.
Bloom, F., Segal, D., Ling, N., and Guillemin, R. (1976). *Science* **194,** 630–632.
Bradbury, A. F., Smyth, D. G., and Snell, C. R. (1976a). *Biochem. Biophys. Res. Commun.* **69,** 950–956.
Bradbury, A. F., Smyth, D. G., and Snell, C. R. (1976b). *Nature (London)* **260,** 793–795.
Brase, D. A., and Sampath-Khanna, S. (1976). *Fed. Proc., Fed. Am. Soc. Exp. Biol.* **35,** 264.
Büscher, H. H., Hill, D. C., Römer, D., Cardinaux, F., Closse, A., Hauser, D., and Pless, J. (1976). *Nature (London)* **261,** 423–425.
Chrétien, M., and Li, C. H. (1967). *Can. J. Biochem.* **45,** 1163–1174.
Chrétien, M., Gilardeau, C., Seidah, N., and Lis, M. (1976a). *Can. J. Biochem.* **54,** 778–782.
Chrétien, M., Benjannet, S., Dragon, N., Seidah, N. G., and Lis, M. (1976b). *Biochem. Biophys. Res. Commun.* **72,** 472–478.
Chrétien, M., Gilardeau, C., Seidah, N., and Lis, M. (1976c). *Canad. J. Biochem.* **54,** 778–782.
Contreras, E., Tomayo, L., Quijada, L., and Silva, E. (1973). *Eur. J. Pharmacol.* **22,** 339–343.
Cox, B. M., Goldstein, A., and Li, C. H. (1976). *Proc. Natl. Acad. Sci. U. S. A.* **73,** 1821–1823.
Cseh, G., Gráf, L., and Goth, F. (1968). *FEBS Lett.* **2,** 42–44.
D'Amour, R. E., and Smith, D. L. (1941). *J. Pharmacol. Exp. Ther.* **72,** 74–79.
Dewey, W. L., Harris, L. S., Howes, J. F., and Nuite, J. D. (1970). *J. Pharmacol. Exp. Ther.* **175,** 435–442.
Doneen, B. A., Chung, D., Yamashiro, D., Law, P. Y., Loh, H. H., and Li, C. H. (1977). *Biochem. Biophys. Res. Commun.* **74,** 656–662.

Dupont, A., Cusan, L., Garon, M., Labrie, F., and Li, C. H. (1977a). *Proc. Natl. Acad. Sci. U. S. A.* **74,** 358–359.

Dupont, A., Cusan, L., Labrie, F., Coy, D. H., and Li, C. H. (1977b). *Biochem. Biophys. Res. Commun.* **75,** 76–82.

Ferland, L., Labrie, F., Coy, D. H., Arimura, A., and Schally, A. V. (1976a). *J. Mol. Cell. Endocrinol.* **4,** 79–88.

Ferland, L., Labrie, F., Jobin, M., Arimura, A., and Schally, A. V. (1976b). *Biochem. Biophys. Res. Commun.* **68,** 149–156.

Ferland, L., Labrie, F., Arimura, A., and Schally, A. V. (1977). *J. Mol. Cell. Endocrinol.* (in press).

Geschwind, I. I., Li, C. H., and Barnafi, L. (1957). *J. Am. Chem. Soc.* **79,** 6394–6401.

Gilardeau, C., and Chrétien, M. (1972). *In* "Chemistry and Biology of Peptides" (J. Meienhofer, ed.), pp. 609–611. Ann Arbor Sci. Publ., Ann Arbor, Michigan.

Gilardeau, G., and Chrétien, M. (1970). *Can. J. Biochem.* **48,** 1017–1021.

Gisin, B. F. (1972). *Anal. Chim. Acta* **58,** 248–249.

Goldstein, A., Lowney, L. I., and Pal, B. K. (1971). *Proc. Natl. Acad. Sci. U. S. A.* **68,** 1742–1747.

Goldstein, A., Goldstein, J. S., and Cox, B. M. (1976). *Life Sci.* **17,** 1643–1654.

Gráf, L., and Cseh, G. (1968). *Biochim. Biophys. Acta* **148,** 175–177.

Gráf, L., and Kenessey, A. (1976). *FEBS Lett.* **69,** 255–260.

Gráf, L., and Li, C. H. (1973). *Biochem. Biophys. Res. Commun.* **53,** 1304–1309.

Gráf, L., Barat, E., Cseh, G., and Sajco, M. (1971). *Biochim. Biophys. Acta* **229,** 276–278.

Gráf, L., Barat, E., and Patthy, A. (1976a). *Acta Biochim. Biophys. Acad. Sci. Hung.* **11,** 121–122.

Gráf, L., Ronai, A. Z., Bajusz, S., Cseh, G., and Székely, J. I. (1976b). *FEBS Lett.* **64,** 181–184.

Gráf, L., Székely, J. I., Ronai, A. Z., Dunai-Kovacs, Z., and Bajusz, S. (1976c). *Nature (London)* **263,** 240–242.

Hagenmaier, H., and Frank, H. (1972). *Hoppe-Seyler's Z. Physiol. Chem.* **353,** 1973–1976.

Haley, T. J., and McCormick, W. G. (1957). *Br. J. Pharmacol. Chemother.* **12,** 12–15.

Hambrook, J. M., Morgan, B. A., Rance, M. J., and Smith, C. F. C. (1976). *Nature (London)* **262,** 782–783.

Hamilton, T. H. (1968). *Science* **161,** 649–661.

Harris, J. I. (1959). *Nature (London)* **184,** 167–169.

Harris, L. S., and Pierson, A. K. (1964). *J. Pharmacol. Exp. Ther.* **143,** 141–148.

Hemmasi, B., and Bayer, E. (1974). *Hoppe-Seyler's Z. Physiol. Chem.* **355,** 481–489.

Herscowitz, H. B., and McKillip, T. W. (1974). *J. Immunol. Methods* **4,** 253–262.

Holaday, J., Loh, H. H., and Li, C. H. (1977). In preparation.

Hosobuchi, Y., Meglio, M., Adams, J. E., and Li, C. H. (1977). *Proc. Natl. Acad. Sci. U.S.A.* **74,** (in press).

Howes, J. F., Harris, L. S., and Dewey, W. L. (1970). *Arch. Int. Pharmacodyn. Ther.* **184,** 267–276.

Hughes, J. (1975). *Brain Res.* **88,** 1–14.

Hughes, J., Smith, T. W., Kosterlitz, H. W., Fothergill, L. A., Morgan, B. A., and Morris, H. R. (1975). *Nature (London)* **258,** 577–579.

Jacquet, Y. F., and Marks, N. (1976). *Science* **194,** 632–635.

Jacquet, Y. F., Marks, N., and Li, C. H. (1976). *In* "Opiates and Endogenous Opioid Peptides" (Kosterlitz, ed.), pp. 411–414. Elsevier, Amsterdam.

Jhamandas, K., Horn, F., and Sutak, M. (1975). *Can. J. Physiol. Pharmacol.* **53,** 540–548.

Kokka, N., Garcia, J. F., George, R., and Elliott, H. W. (1972). *Endocrinology* **90,** 735–743.

Konig, W., and Geiger, R. (1970). *Chem. Ber.* **103,** 788–798.
Koster, R., Anderson, M., and DeBeer, E. J. (1959). *Fed. Proc., Fed. Am. Soc. Exp. Biol.* **18,** 412.
Kosterlitz, H. W., Lydon, R. J., and Watt, A. J. (1970). *Br. J. Pharmacol.* **39,** 398–413.
Lazarus, L. H., Ling, N., and Guillemin, R. (1976). *Proc. Natl. Acad. Sci. U. S. A.* **73,** 2156–2159.
Lee, N. M., Loh, H. H., and Li, C. H. (ms. in prep).
Li, C. H. (1964). *Nature (London)* **201,** 924.
Li, C. H., and Chung, D. (1976a). *Proc. Natl. Acad. Sci. U. S. A.* **73,** 1145–1148.
Li, C. H., and Chung, D. (1976b). *Nature (London)* **260,** 622–624.
Li, C. H., Barnafi, L., Chrétien, M., and Chung, D. (1965). *Nature (London)* **208,** 1093–1094.
Li, C. H., Barnafi, L., Chrétien, M., and Chung, D. *Proc. Pan-Am. Congr. Endocrinol., 6th, 1966* Excerpta Med. Found. Int. Congr. Ser. No. 112, pp. 334–364.
Li, C. H., Danho, W. O., Chung, D., and Rao, A. J. (1975). *Biochemistry* **14,** 947–952.
Li, C. H., Lemaire, S., Yamashiro, D., and Doneen, B. A. (1976a). *Biochem. Biophys. Res. Commun.* **71,** 19–25.
Li, C. H., Chung, D., and Doneen, B. A. (1976b). *Biochem. Biophys. Res. Commun.* **72,** 1542–1547.
Li, C. H., Yamashiro, D., Tseng, L. F., and Loh, H. H. (1977a). *J. Med. Chem.* **20,** 325–328.
Li, C. H., Rao, A. J., Doneen, B. A., and Yamashiro, D. (1977b). *Biochem. Biophys. Res. Commun.* **75,** 576–580.
Li, C. H., Yamashiro, D., Tseng, L. F., and Loh, H. H. (1977c). *Int. J. Pept. Prot. Res.* **10,** (in press).
Ling, N., Burgus, R., and Guillemin, R. (1976). *Proc. Natl. Acad. Sci. U.S.A.* **73,** 3942–3946.
Litchfield, J. T., and Wilcoxon, F. (1949). *J. Pharmacol. Exp. Ther.* **96,** 99–113.
Loh, H. H., Tseng, L. F., Wei, E., and Li, C. H. (1976). *Proc. Natl. Acad. Sci. U. S. A.* **73,** 2895–2896.
Lohmar, P., and Li, C. H. (1967). *Biochim. Biophys. Acta* **147,** 381–383.
Matthews, J. D., Labrecque, G., and Domino, E. F. (1973). *Psychopharmacologia* **29,** 113–120.
Meglio, M., Hosobuchi, Y., Loh, H. H., Adams, J. E., and Li, C. H. (1977). *Proc. Natl. Acad. Sci. U. S. A.* **74,** 774–776.
Meites, J. (1966). *In* "Neuroendocrinology" (L. Martini and W. F. Ganong, eds.), Vol. 1, pp. 669–707. Academic Press, New York.
Merrifield, R. B. (1963). *J. Am. Chem. Soc.* **85,** 2149–2154.
Montel, H., Starke, K., and Weber, F. (1974). *Naunyn-Schmiedeberg's Arch. Pharmacol.* **283,** 357–369.
Pankov, Y. A., and Yudeau, M. A. (1972). *Biokhimiya* **37,** 991–1031.
Pasternak, G. W., Goodman, R., and Snyder, S. H. (1975). *Life Sci.* **16,** 1765–1769.
Pert, C. B., and Snyder, S. H. (1973). *Science* **179,** 1011–1014.
Pert, C. B., Aposhian, D., and Snyder, S. H. (1975). *Brain Res.* **75,** 112–116.
Pert, C. B., Pert, A., Chang, J. K., and Fong, B. T. W. (1976). *Science* **194,** 330–332.
Pickering, B. T., and Li, C. H. (1963). *Biochim. Biophys. Acta* **74,** 156–157.
Rivier, C., Vale, W., Ling, N., Brown, M., and Guillemin, R. (1977). *Endocrinology* **100,** 238–241.
Saarnivaara, L. (1969). *Ann. Med. Exp. Biol. Fenn.* **47,** 113–123.
Sampath-Khanna, S., Brase, D. A., Loh, H. H., and Way, E. L. (1977). In press.
Scott, A. P., and Lowry, P. J. (1974). *Biochem. J.* **139,** 593–602.

Simantov, R., and Snyder, S. H. (1976a). *Life Sci.* **18,** 781–788.
Simantov, R., and Snyder, S. H. (1976b). *Proc. Natl. Acad. Sci. U. S. A.* **73,** 2515–2519.
Simon, E. J., Hiller, J. M., and Edelman, I. (1973). *Proc. Natl. Acad. Sci. U.S.A.* **70,** 1947–1949.
Snyder, S. H. (1975). *Nature (London)* **257,** 185–189.
Tata, J. R. (1970). *In* "Biochemical Actions of Hormones" (G. Litwac, ed.), Vol. 1, p. 89. Academic Press, New York.
Terenius, L. (1973). *Acta Pharmacol. Toxicol.* **33,** 377–384.
Terenius, L., and Wahlström, A. (1975). *Life Sci.* **16,** 1759–1764.
Tilis, G., Hickey, J., and Guyda, H. (1975). *J. Clin. Endocrinol. Metabl.* **41,** 797–800.
Tomayo, L., and Contreras, E. (1965). *Arch. Biol. Med. Exp.* **2,** 70.
Tseng, L. F., Loh, H. H., and Li, C. H. (1977). *Biochem. Biophys. Res. Commun.* **74,** 390–396.
Waterfield, A. A., Hughes, J., and Kosterlitz, H. W. (1976). *Nature (London)* **260,** 624–625.
Way, E. L., Loh, H. H., and Shen, F. H. (1969). *J. Pharmacol. Exp. Ther.* **167,** 1–8.
Way, E. L., Ho, I. K., and Loh, H. H. (1974). *Adv. Biochem. Psychopharmacol.* **10,** 219–231.
Wei, E., and Loh, H. H. (1976). *Science* **193,** 1262–1263.
Yamashiro, D., and Li, C. H. (1973). *J. Am. Chem. Soc.* **95,** 1310–1315.
Yamashiro, D., and Li, C. H. (1974). *Proc. Natl. Acad. Sci. U. S. A.,* **71,** 4945–4949.
Yamashiro, D., Blake, J., and Li, C. H. (1976). *Tetrahedron Lett.*, 1469–1472.
Yamashiro, D., Tseng, L. F., Doneen, B. A., Loh, H. H., and Li, C. H. (1977). *Int. J. Pept. Prot. Res.* **10,** 159–166.
Yudeau, M. A., and Pankov, Y. A. (1970). *Probl. Endocrinol.* **16,** 49–51.

3

Lipotropins

M. CHRÉTIEN AND M. LIS

I. Introduction

Interest in the role of pituitary hormones in adipose tissue metabolism began many years ago when Anselmino and Hoffman (1931) demonstrated that extracts of anterior pituitaries could produce ketosis. In 1936, Best and Campbell found, repeating these experiments, that such extracts produce body weight loss and hepatic lipid accumulation. Later, when individual hormones were obtained in pure form, it was recognized that adrenocorticotropic hormone (ACTH) and somatotropic hormone (STH) could influence lipid mobilization as reflected in the accumulation of hepatic lipid and the production of ketosis. Preparations of thyrotropin (TSH) were also found to produce ketosis and fatty infiltration of the liver. The demonstration that ACTH stimulates the release of free fatty acids from rat adipose tissue *in vitro* came later in the work of White and Engel (1958). They found that some preparations of growth hormone also exhibit lipolytic activities *in vitro,* although compared to ACTH, high levels of these preparations are required to obtain a similar response. Later investigations with TSH purified from various sources indicated that this hormone also possesses an intrinsic lipolytic activity as measured *in vitro* and that it is not acting only in relation to stimulation of thyroid hormone secretion (Freinkel, 1961; Rudman *et al.,* 1963).

Given the observation that the N-terminal segment 1–17 of ACTH exhibits lipolytic activity *in vitro* (Tanaka *et al.,* 1962), it is not surprising that the melanocyte-stimulating hormones (α-MSH and β-MSH), and other synthetic peptides structurally related to ACTH (Raben *et al.,* 1961; Rudman *et al.,* 1963) also possess the same *in vitro* lipolytic activity.

Rudman and Seidman (1958) found that crude extracts of porcine pituitaries produce gross lipemia when injected into rabbits. He named his newly purified component fraction H. Astwood *et al.* (1961) isolated two similar peptides (peptide I and peptide II) from porcine pituitaries. Since 1964, Li and his group (Li, 1964; Li *et al.,* 1965, 1966; Chrétien and Li, 1967a,b; Lohmar and Li, 1967) have published a series of articles on new substances isolated from ovine and bovine pituitaries. They were named ovine α-, β-, and γ-LPH, and this terminology has been used for the identification of similar material from the pituitaries of other species.

Gilardeau and Chrétien (1970a,b), Gráf and Cseh (1968), Gráf *et al.* (1969), and Yudaev and Pankov (1970) have isolated and characterized similar substances from porcine pituitary glands. These factors differ from those of Rudman *et al.* (1970), Astwood *et al.* (1961), Friesen (1964), Schleyer *et al.* (1969a,b), and Schwandt *et al.* (1968, 1969) who repeated some of Rudman's experiments. Trygstad (1965, 1967, 1968; Trygstad and Foss, 1967) and Leites and Davtyan (1963, 1965a,b) have also tried to purify similar substances from human pituitaries. Rishka and Khokhlov (1965) have purified a lipolytic substance from pituitaries of different species and found that it has methionine at the N-terminus, thus it differs from the other known hypophyseal hormones. Finally, Smith *et al.* (1975)

and Gráf *et al.* (1974) have isolated two lipolytic hormones from human pituitary glands, which again differ from the above lipotropins since they are lacking tryptophan. Moreover, both are different from each other, since they have different N-terminal groups and different amino acid compositions.

Several other groups, employing different purification methods, have isolated pituitary fractions believed to contain lipolytic peptides. Burns *et al.* (1967) showed that certain fractions of human growth hormone (HGH) preparations possess lipolytic activity on human adipose tissue *in vitro*. Leites and Davtyan (1963, 1965a,b) isolated a lipolytic substance (adiposin) from ox and pig pituitaries. This substance is active in the rabbit, rat, and human adipose tissue. Further, Abdurakhmanov and Lipovetzky (1966) isolated from human pituitaries a lipid-mobilizing factor (LMF), which produces hyperlipemia and hypercholesterolemia. The structural characteristics of the peptides isolated by Leites and Davtyan (1963), Trygstad (1965), Burns *et al.* (1967), and most of the others were not sufficiently determined to permit structural comparison.

Li *et al.* (1965), Chrétien and Li (1967a,b), and Lohmar and Li (1967) were the first to determine the complete sequence of their compounds (β-LPH from ox pituitaries, β- and γ-LPH from sheep). More recently, Gráf and Cseh (1968), Gráf *et al.* (1969), and Gilardeau and Chrétien (1970a,b) completed the purification and chemical characterization of β- and γ-LPH from pig pituitaries.

II. Purification

A. β-LPH (Ovine, Bovine, Porcine, and Human)

These four β-LPH's were purified essentially by the method of Li *et al.* (1965), with some modifications. The stage of purification by means of the ion-exchange resin IRC-50, was, for example, replaced by carboxymethyl cellulose (CM cellulose), under different conditions in the case of porcine β-LPH (Gilardeau and Chrétien, 1970a). The basic procedure was as follows: extraction with acid acetone, precipitation with NaCl, and dialysis at 0° (Fig. 1). During dialysis, a precipitate forms and is removed by centrifugation. The clear supernatant was lyophilized (fraction D). This fraction was then chromatographed on CM cellulose stabilized with a 0.01 *M* ammonium acetate buffer at pH 4.6. The elution gradient (pH and buffer concentration) was obtained as described by Birk and Li (1964).

One of the peaks was identified as corresponding to β-LPH (Fig. 2). This fraction was lyophilized three times to remove the ammonium ace-

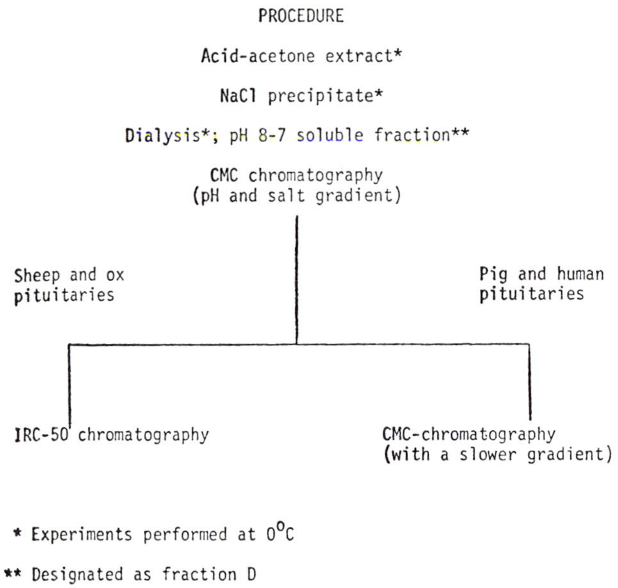

FIG. 1. Steps in the isolation of β-LPH from human, sheep, ox, and pig pituitary glands.

tate and run on an IRC-50 column or again on CMC under slightly modified conditions to yield pure β-LPH.

The extreme rarity of the starting material rendered purification of human LPH's difficult. Schwandt *et al.* (1968, 1969), nevertheless, has identified a human fraction H, and Cseh *et al.* (1968, 1972), using glands preserved with acetone, and Chrétien (1973), using fresh frozen glands,

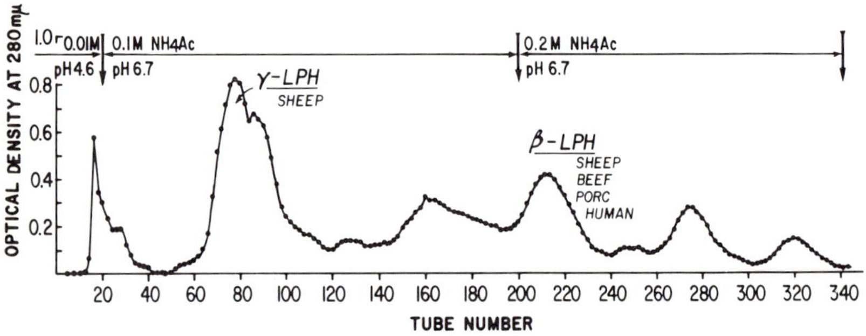

FIG. 2. Chromatography on CM cellulose of various compounds purified from pituitaries of different species. The initial buffer used was composed of 0.01 *M* ammonium acetate at pH 4.6. At the twentieth tube, a gradient is produced by gradually increasing the saline concentration and raising the pH. A solution of ammonium acetate 0.1 *M* at pH 6.7 is added to the initial buffer contained in a 500-ml Erlenmeyer flask. At tube 200, an 0.2 *M* solution is added.

were able to purify human lipolytic hormones. The material from these last two groups is analogous, but not fully identical (Chrétien, 1973), possibly because that the preparations were not absolutely pure.

B. γ-LPH (Ovine)

To obtain analytically pure γ-LPH, the procedures for purification of β-LPH (Fig. 1) were used in part. As the γ-LPH molecule has a more acid isoelectric point, it is eluted from CMC before β-LPH (Fig. 2). Two further purification stages, therefore, were necessary. The DEAE cellulose was equilibrated with 0.0075 *M* ammonium acetate buffer (pH 7.0), and the elution was performed with a gradient made by introducing 0.175 *M* ammonium acetate (pH 7.0) through a 500-ml mixing flask. The fractions collected were lyophilized several times to remove water and ammonium acetate. Peak C_2, which was the most active, was rechromatographed on DEAE cellulose under identical conditions.

The main peak obtained from the second DEAE cellulose chromatography step was applied to a small column (1 × 15 cm) of CM cellulose equilibrated with 0.01 *M* ammonium acetate buffer of pH 4.6. Stepwise elution was carried out with increasing concentrations (0.01–0.035 *M*) of ammonium acetate at a constant pH of 4.6. This material was pure on polyacrylamide gel electrophoresis, amino acid analysis, and ultracentrifugation studies, and its structure was determined.

III. Structure Studies

As shown in Table I, it is evident that the pituitary glands contain a variety of lipolytic peptides. Rudman's substance may be similar to the neurophysins, as well as the peptides of Preddie and Saffran (1965), and of Wuu and Saffran (1969). They are considered to be from the neurohypophysis. On the other hand, Li *et al.* (1966), Chrétien and Li (1967a,b), and Lohmar and Li (1967) have completed the chemical characterization of bovine and ovine β-LPH and of γ-LPH. Gráf and Cseh (1968), Gráf *et al.* (1969), and Gilardeau and Chrétien (1970a,b, 1972) have published the complete characterization of porcine β-LPH. Finally, Smith (1973), Smith *et al.* (1975), and Gráf *et al.* (1974) have recently described the isolation of two different lipolytic hormones from human glands. These two new substances differ from the well-characterized lipotropins because both are lacking tryptophan. Moreover, both are different from each other, since they do not possess the same N-terminal group and have marked differences in their amino acid compositions.

TABLE I—Amino Acid Composition of Different Lipolytic Hormones

Amino Acid	Residues/molecule					Human β-LPH		Human lipolytic peptide	
	Ovine β-LPH	Ovine γ-LPH	Bovine β-LPH	Porcine β-LPH	Porcine γ-LPH	Czeh	Chrétien	Smith	Gráf 1
Lys	11	4	10	10	4	10	8	14.8	3.2
His	2	1	2	2	1	2	2	15.5	1.1
Arg	5	4	5	4	3	5	6	5.6	4.0
Asp	4	2	4	5	3	9	8	8.0	6.2
Thr	4	1	4	3	0	4	4	1.7	2.8
Ser	5	3	5	3	1	5	6	5.0	3.7
Glu	16	13	17	14	11	13	14	3.6	11.0
Pro	5	4	5	9	8	6	6	6.0	4.6
Gly	8	5	8	8	5	9	8	8.4	7.8
Ala	13	11	14	15	13	8	6	10.9	5.8
$\frac{1}{2}$ Cys	0	0	0	0	0	0	0	0	5.5
Val	2	1	2	3	1	3	4	10.0	1.6
Met	2	1	2	2	1	2	2	0	0.7
Ileu	1	0	1	1	0	2	2	0.32	1.0
Leu	6	4	6	5	3	7	8	7.9	5.1
Tyr	3	2	3	3	2	3	2	1.3	0.9
Phe	3	1	3	3	1	3	4	1.4	2.7
Trp	1	1	1	1	1	1	Not determined	0	
	91	58	92	91	58	92	≥90		

There is some evidence that Astwood's peptide I and Chrétien's γ-LPH might be similar, since their molecular weights are almost identical, and their C-terminal segments have the same amino acid sequence (Hoffmann and Katsoyannis, 1963). There are indications (Rudman *et al.,* 1970; Schleyer *et al.,* 1969a,b) that fraction H, peptide II, and Schleyer's peptide are markedly different from β- and γ-LPH, although the chemical characterization is incomplete. It is evident that Rudman's peptides are more closely related to peptide II (Astwood *et al.,* 1961; Friesen, 1964), the peptides of Preddie and Saffran (1965) and Wuu and Saffran (1969) and to Hollenberg's neurophysins (Hollenberg and Hope, 1968; Rauch *et al.,* 1969) than to β- and γ-LPH. Tryptophan is present and half-cystine is absent in ACTH, α- and β-MSH, β- and γ-LPH, while in Rudman's fractions the former is absent, and the latter is present.

We will consider mainly the chemical structure of the lipotropic peptides that have been well characterized. Figure 3 shows that ovine β-LPH consists of 91 amino acid and has a molecular weight (MW) of 9958.

The segment 41–58 is identical to the complete structure of β-MSH, thus containing the particular sequence Met-Glu-His-Phe-Arg-Trp-Gly, which is present at the active center of α- and β-MSH and ACTH (Li, 1964; Li *et al.,* 1965, 1966). It is important to note that immediately before and immediately after the site of the cleavage postulated in β-LPH to yield β-MSH, there are two diamino acids. Further, we recently showed that pig pituitaries also produce a β-LPH which, in the interior of its molecule, carries the amino acid sequence of pig β-MSH (Fig. 3).

Bovine β-LPH (Lohmar and Li, 1967) has the same amino acid composition and the same N-terminal amino acid and is believed to have a structure identical to ovine β-LPH. On the other hand, porcine β-LPH has significant differences in its proline content and in its isoelectric point (porcine β-LPH 6.43; ovine β-LPH 8.30) (Gilardeau and Chrétien, 1970b, 1972; Gráf *et al.,* 1969). The sequence was determined using a combination of manual and automatic Edman degradation.

It was applied to the whole molecule of β-LPH and to its cyanogen bromide (CNBr) fragments. Their amino acid compositions of CNBr fragments are presented in Table II. Peptide I has the same NH_2-terminal amino acid as the entire molecule, glutamic acid, and corresponds to amino acid 1–47. Peptides III and V do not contain homoserine, and, thus, they must be the COOH-terminal. V minus III gives the amino acid composition of peptide IV; thus, the fragments must be arranged I-IV-III. Peptides II and V are overlaps.

The first 45 amino acid residues were identified by sequencing the whole molecule of β-LPH; residues 39–40, however, did not give any results and were deduced from the amino acid composition of segment 1–47. This

γ-LPH	Glu-Leu-...-Lys-Lys-Asp-Ser-Gly-Pro-Tyr-Lys-Met-Glu-His-Phe-Arg-Try-Gly-Ser-Pro-Pro-Lys-Asp
Sheep	1 2 39 40 41 42 43 44 45 46 47 48 49 50 51 52 53 54 55 56 57 58
β-LPH	Glu-Leu-...-Lys-Lys-Asp-Ser-Gly-Pro-Tyr-Lys-Met-Glu-His-Phe-Arg-Try-Gly-Ser-Pro-Pro-Lys-Asp-Lys-Arg-...-Gl
Sheep	1 2 39 40 41 42 43 44 45 46 47 48 49 50 51 52 53 54 55 56 57 58 59 60 91
Ox	
β-MSH	Asp-Ser-Gly-Pro-Tyr-Lys-Met-Glu-His-Phe-Arg-Try-Gly-Ser-Pro-Pro-Lys-Asp
Ox	1 2 3 4 5 6 7 8 9 10 11 12 13 14 15 16 17 18
Sheep	
β-LPH	Glu-Leu-...-Lys-Lys-Asp-Glu-Gly-Pro-Tyr-Lys-Met-Glu-His-Phe-Arg-Try-Gly-Ser-Pro-Pro-Lys-Asp-Lys-Arg-...-Gl
Pig	1 2 39 40 41 42 43 44 45 46 47 48 49 50 51 52 53 54 55 56 57 58 59 60 91
γ-LPH	Glu-Leu-... Asp-Glu-Gly-Pro-Tyr-Lys-Met-Glu-His-Phe-Arg-Try-Gly-Ser-Pro-Pro-Lys-Asp
Pig	1 2 41 42 43 44 45 46 47 48 49 50 51 52 53 54 55 56 57 58
β-MSH	Asp-Glu-Gly-Pro-Tyr-Lys-Met-Glu-His-Phe-Arg-Try-Gly-Ser-Pro-Pro-Lys-Asp
Pig	1 2 3 4 5 6 7 8 9 10 11 12 13 14 15 16 17 18

FIG. 3. Comparison of the structures of melanocyte-stimulating hormones and lipotropic hormones.

segment shows that there are still 3 lysines to be placed in the first 46 residues. These 3 lysines must be at positions 39, 40, and 46. This gives the sequence of the first 47 amino acids residues, methionine being the forty-seventh.

The Edman degradation of peptide II with dimethylallylamine buffer gave the sequence 48–54. And peptides V and III gave, respectively, the sequences 48–64 and 66–83, except residues 79 and 80, which were not identifiable. From the amino acid composition of peptide IV, methionine must be at position 65. The remaining residues were placed after enzymatic studies of fragments.

The digestion of peptide III with chymotrypsin yielded two main products after purification by paper electrophoresis in collidine–acetate buffer and paper chromatography in *n*-butanol, pyridine, acetic acid, and water (90:60:18:72), as shown in Table III. Peptide C1 corresponds to residues 66–78, the sequence of which is already known; and peptide C2 to residues 79–91. This last peptide contains four lysines and has a lysine at its NH_2-terminus, as determined by dansylation. It was digested with trypsin, and gave, as shown in Table IV, the peptides needed to establish the complete sequence of porcine β-LPH.

TABLE II—Amino Acid Analysis of Porcine β-LPH Fragments after Cleavage with Cyanogen Bromide

Amino acid	No. of residues/molecule					
	I (1–47)	IV (48–65)	II (1–65)	III (66–91)	V (48–91)	LPH
Ser	1	1	1	0	0	0
Trp	0	1	1	0	1	1
Lys	3.1 (3)	2.1 (2)	4.9 (5)	5.0 (5)	6.8 (7)	10
His	0	0.9 (1)	1.0 (1)	1.1 (1)	1.8 (2)	2
Arg	1.9 (2)	1.8 (2)	3.7 (4)	0	1.7 (2)	4
Asp	2.3 (2)	1.0 (1)	3.2 (3)	2.0 (2)	3.1 (3)	5
Thr	0.1 (0)	0.1 (0)	0.1 (0)	2.7 (3)	2.8 (3)	3
Ser	0	0.9 (1)	1.2 (1)	1.8 (2)	2.7 (3)	3
Glu	10.2 (10)	1.3 (1)	11.3 (11)	2.9 (3)	4.1 (4)	14
Pro	6.2 (6)	1.8 (2)	7.8 (8)	0.6 (1)	2.8 (3)	9
Gly	3.4 (4)	2.6 (3)	6.8 (7)	1.0 (1)	4.1 (4)	8
Ala	12.6 (13)	0.1 (0)	12.9 (13)	2.0 (2)	2.2 (2)	15
½ Cys	0	0	0	0	0	0
Val	1.0 (1)	0.03 (0)	0.8 (1)	1.7 (2)	1.6 (2)	3
Met	0	0	0.5 (1)	0	0.5 (1)	2
Ile	0.07 (0)	0.01 (0)	0.05 (0)	0.5 (1)	0.6 (1)	1
Leu	2.9 (3)	0.05 (0)	2.8 (3)	1.7 (2)	1.9 (2)	5
Tyr	1.7 (2)	0.85 (1)	2.7 (3)	0.05 (0)	0.9 (1)	3
Phe	0.05 (0)	1.9 (2)	1.9 (2)	1.0 (1)	2.9 (3)	3
	47	18	65	26	44	91

Peptide C2T2 (80–84) has the sequence Asn-Ala-Ile-Val-Lys, since Ala-Ile-Val were already placed by the sequencer on BrCN fragment III, and since Asn was found to be the NH_2-terminal residue from dansylation and leucine amino peptidase digestion.

Only residues 85–91 remain unknown. These correspond to peptides C2T1 and C2T3. Results are summarized in Table IV. Although C2T1 is a tryptic peptide, it contains two lysine residues. The NH_2-terminal residue, as determined by dansylation, is aspartic acid. Leucine aminopeptidase cleaved mainly Asn and Ala after 8 hours of incubation. This sequence must be Asn-Ala-(His-Lys)-Lys.

The COOH-terminal residue of β-LPH, as determined by carboxypeptidase A digestions, is glutamine. Equimolecular amounts of glycine and lysine were also released in much smaller quantities than glutamine. Since peptide C2T3 contains Gly-Glu, the COOH-terminus must be Lys-Gly-Gln; and since there is almost no histidine release by carboxypeptidase A, there must be two consecutive lysines at positions 88 and 89.

From these data, the following sequence is proposed:

5 10 15 20
Glu-Leu-Ala-Gly- Ala-Pro-Pro-Glu-Pro- Ala-Arg-Asp-Pro-Glu- Ala-Pro-Ala-Glu-Gly- Ala-
25 30 35 40
Ala-Ala-Arg-Ala-Glu -Leu-Glu-Tyr-Gly- Leu -Val-Ala-Glu-Ala- Glu -Ala-Ala-Glu-Lys- Lys -
45 50 55 60
Asp-Glu-Gly-Pro- Tyr -Lys-Met-Glu-His- Phe -Arg-Trp Gly-Ser- Pro-Pro-Lys-Asp-Lys- Arg-
65 70 75 80
Tyr-Gly-Gly-Phe- Met-Thr-Ser-Glu-Lys- Ser -Gln-Thr-Pro-Leu- Val -Thr-Leu-Phe-Lys- Asn -
85 90
Ala-Ile-Val-Lys- Asn -Ala-His-Lys-Lys- Gly -Gln

The sequence reported here is almost identical to the one reported by Gráf *et al*. (1974); for residue 35, we find glutamic acid instead of glutamine. They use the Edman dansyl methodology on a chymotryptic peptide from residue 29 to 45 to determine this amino acid. Since the mobilities of the dansyl peptides were not published, it is impossible to understand what happened.

The C-terminal portion of porcine β-LPH is almost identical to that of ovine β-LPH, while its 43 amino acids from the N-terminus contain more proline residues so that the amino acid sequence is at least slightly differ-

Table III—Amino Acid Compositions of Fragments from Chymotryptic Cleavage of Peptide 66–91

Amino acid	No. of residues/molecule			
	C 1	C 2	C 1 + C 2	Peptide 66–91
Trp	0	0	0	0
Lys	1.0 (1)	4.1 (4)	5	5
His	0	1.0 (1)	1	1
Arg	0	0	0	0
Asp	0	1.9 (2)	2	2
Thr	2.6 (3)	0	3	3
Ser	1.7 (2)	0	2	2
Glu	1.9 (2)	0.9 (1)	3	3
Pro	1.0 (1)	0	1	1
Gly	0.1 (0)	0.9 (1)	1	1
Ala	0	1.8 (2)	2	2
Val	1.0 (1)	0.8 (1)	2	2
Met	0	0	0	0
Ile	0	0.5 (1)	1	1
Leu	1.7 (2)	0	2	2
Tyr	0	0	0	0
Phe	0.6 (1)	0	1	1
	13	13	26	26

TABLE IV—Amino Acid Sequence of Segment 79–91 of Porcine β-LPH

Segment	Method used	Sequence
C2	Dansylation	Lys-(Asn, Ala, Ile, Val, Lys, Asn, Ala, His, Lys, Lys, Gly, Gln)
C2T1	Dansylation + LAP	Asn- Ala-(His, Lys)-Lys
C2T2	Dansylation + LAP	Asn- (Ala, Ile, Val)- Lys
C2T3	Dansylation	Gly- Gln
C2T4		Lys
β-LPH	Carboxypeptidase A	Lys- Lys-Gly- Gln
Fragment IV from BrCN cleavage	Edman degradation	---(Lys, Asn)- Ala- Ile- Val- (Lys- Asn, Ala, His, Lys, Lys, Gly, Gln)
Proposed sequence		Lys- Asn- Ala- Ile- Val- Lys- Asn- Ala- His- Lys- Lys-Gly- Gln 79 80 81 82 83 84 85 86 87 88 89 90 91

end (Gilardeau and Chrétien, 1970a,b, 1972). Table V shows the 10 differences in amino acid sequence between ovine and porcine β-LPH.

The chemical structure of ovine γ-LPH has been determined (Chrétien and Li, 1967a,b). It has 58 amino acids and an MW of approximately 6500 (Chrétien and Li, 1967a,b). γ-LPH has the same amino acid sequence as segment 1–58 of β-LPH. Figure 3 shows these similarities and includes the structure of porcine β-LPH as determined by Gilardeau and Chrétien (1970a,b, 1972).

IV. β-MSH Precursor Hypothesis

The discovery of γ-LPH by Chrétien and Li (1967a,b) appeared unique in that, for the first time, a compound had been found possessing a structure that could be considered an intermediary product between two other known substances. β-LPH and β-MSH (Fig. 3). At that time, we proposed three hypotheses: (a) that the pituitary synthesizes *de novo* a series of peptides containing, in part, an identical sequence; (b) that a large molecule is formed and later split into smaller fragments in the pituitary cells; (c) that β-LPH is degraded during the isolation process.

At the same time, Steiner *et al*. (1967) published an article demonstrating that insulin was synthesized from a larger and relatively inactive precursor called proinsulin. These findings resulted from incorporation experiments and chase labeling *in vitro* in tissue slices incubated in the presence of radioactive amino acids. The same experimental approach has been used for parathormone (Cohn *et al.,* 1972; Habener *et al.,* 1972, 1973; Kemper *et al.,* 1972) and glucagon (Rigopoulou *et al.,* 1970; Noe and Bauer 1971, 1973; Tager and Steiner, 1973), which are also synthesized in the form of precursors.

TABLE V—Differences between Ovine and Porcine β-LPH

Residue	Ovine	Porcine
3	Thr	Ala
5	Glu	Ala
6	Arg	Pro
7	Leu	Pro
9	Gln	Pro
12	Gly	Asp
16	Gln	Pro
19	Ser	Gly
42	Ser	Glu
83	Ile	Val

Chrétien and Gilardeau (1970) showed that β-LPH is not broken down chemically or enzymatically during the isolation process, for the intermediate product, γ-LPH, was present in hypophyseal extracts when less rigorous extraction conditions were employed. They further demonstrated that β-LPH was highly resistant to vigorous chemical treatment, thereby lessening the probability of degradation during purification. Moreover, it is unlikely that enzymatic breakdown occurs during purification, since all procedures except chromatography on CM cellulose are performed at 0°. Finally, incubation of pituitary powder with a mixture of acetic acid and acetone for 20 minutes at 50° gave a good yield of β-LPH.

Chance *et al.* (1968) had published the complete structure of pig proinsulin, and pointed to the presence of two diamino acids at the cleavage sites (Fig. 4). This resemblance at the cleavage sites to the structure of the LPH peptides was striking, and it became clear that the hypothesis of a biologic precursor stated above was the most probable, i.e., that β-LPH, 100 times less active than β-MSH, was the biologic precursor of the latter, and that γ-LPH was an intermediate component. Further reports (Steiner *et al.,* 1968; Yip, 1968) have indicated that proinsulin, too, is probably transformed into an intermediary substance called double-chain proinsulin before being converted into insulin. These resemblances strongly suggest that the enzymes in the pituitary and the pancreas have similar biologic properties. A model has also been established for proparathormone on this basis (Habener *et al.,* 1973; Kemper *et al.,* 1972). Moreover, the same group has recently shown that there exists a precursor to the proparathyroid hormone, which they called pre-pro-PTH (Kemper *et al.,* 1974).

The precursor model of β-LPH, γ-LPH, and β-MSH has been found in sheep, beef, porcine, and human pituitaries. However, Scott and Lowry (1974) and Bloomfield *et al.* (1974) believe that human β-MSH does not exist as a distinct entity and is a degradation product, but their data are

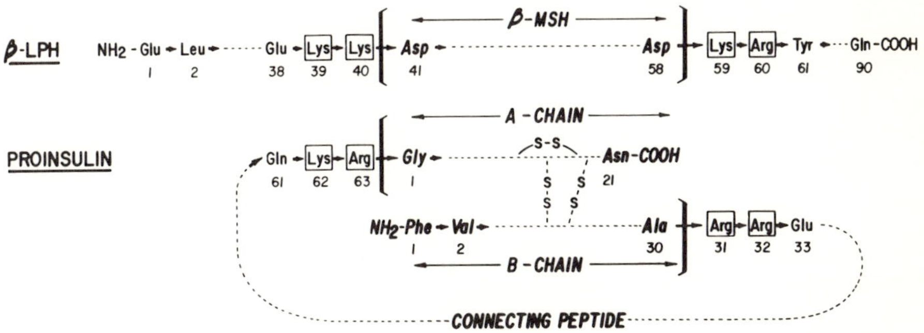

FIG. 4. The amino acid sequences of β-LPH and proinsulin showing the two basic amino acids at the site of enzymatic cleavage.

based on radioimmunoassay after Sephadex separation and do not take into account the fact that the process of transformation of β-LPH into γ-LPH and probably into β-MSH is slow, as we have shown in our biosynthetic studies.

V. *In Vitro* Biosynthesis

A. β-LPH

Our studies on the structure of γ- and β-LPH led us to the same conclusions as those reached by Steiner in his work on the biosynthesis of insulin (Steiner *et al.*, 1967). Chance, with his results on the structure of proinsulin, confirmed our hypothesis of cleavage at the level of the diamino acids (Chance *et al.*, 1968). We, thus, decided to study the biosynthesis of β-LPH using the chase-labeling method (Bertagna *et al.*, 1974). We incubated slices of ox or sheep pituitary with a radioactive amino acid or mixture of amino acids, and purified the biosynthetic radioactive β-LPH by the method of Li *et al.* (1965). We succeeded in demonstrating that these slices of pituitary gland incorporate the labeled amino acids *in vitro*

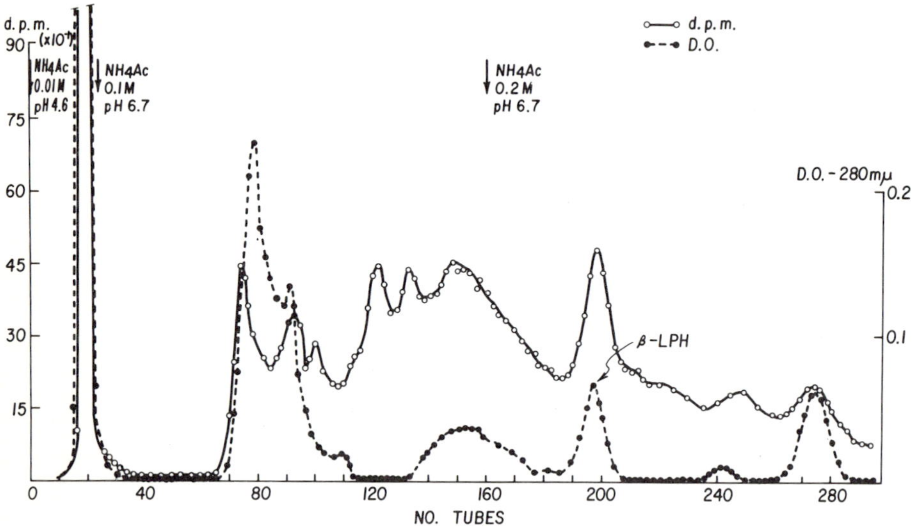

FIG. 5. CM cellulose chromatography of a fraction D. The column was 40 × 1 cm. A continuous gradient was started at tube 20 by the addition of 0.01 *M* NH_4 Ac buffer, pH 6.7, to a 250-ml mixing chamber containing 0.01 *M* buffer pH 4.6. At tube 160, a 0.2 *M* NH_4Ac solution was used to increase the gradient. Fractions of 2 ml were collected at a rate of 1 ml/minute.

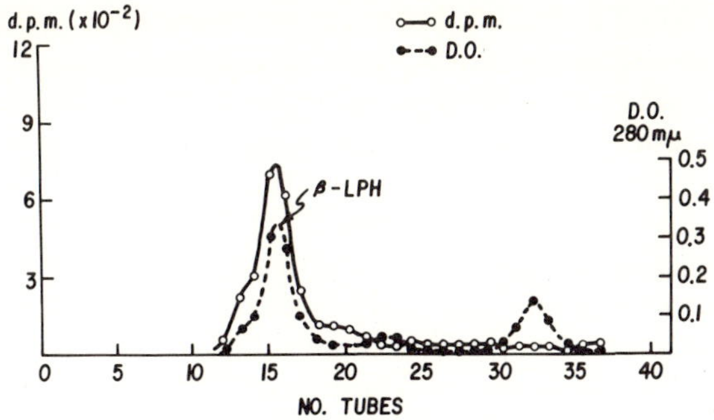

FIG. 6. Chromatography of peaks 192–205 from Fig. 5 on molecular filter Sephadex G-50.

in a material that is inseparable from standard β-LPH, by either ion-exchange resins (CM cellulose) (Fig. 5), molecular filters (Sephadex G-50) (Fig. 6), or electrophoresis on polyacrylamide gel (Fig. 7).

B. γ-LPH

β-LPH occurs in minute amounts in the pituitary, and the newly synthesized radioactive β-LPH constitutes about 1% of the total radioactivity. γ-LPH occurs in still smaller amounts and was more difficult to isolate. Nevertheless, using a modification of an isolation procedure previously described (Bertagna *et al.*, 1974) after incubation of pituitary tissue

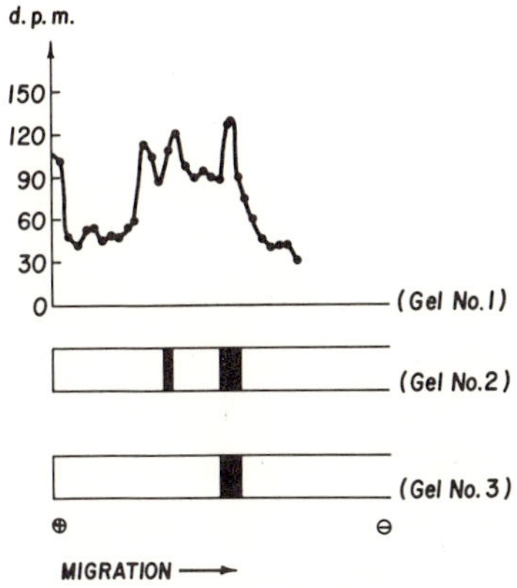

FIG. 7. Electrophoresis on polyacrylamide gel (5.6%) at pH 4.5. An aliquot (1500 dpm/200 μg) of the fraction from the Sephadex G-50 run (Fig. 6) was applied on gel No. 1. The gel was cut into slices and counting carried out. Gel No. 2 has an aliquot identical with that on gel No. 1, but stained only. Standard β-LPH was applied on gel No. 3. Each slice was counted for 20 minutes so as to give a standard deviation of 2.5–4.5%.

with ^{3}H-labeled lysine, we were able to isolate a radioactive protein with all the chemical characteristics of γ-LPH (Chrétien *et al.*, 1975).

In 1974, we were able to demonstrate the biosynthesis of β-LPH in incubations lasting 4 hours (Bertagna *et al.*, 1974). In the subsequent experiments (Chrétien *et al.*, 1975), the incubation was prolonged for 12 hours, and the elution pattern of radioactive proteins from CM cellulose was different. Radioactive β-LPH was absent, and the main peak of radioactivity was in the γ-LPH region (Fig. 8). This could be interpreted as an indication that β-LPH is transformed into γ-LPH. The identification of newly synthesized radioactive γ-LPH was done by elution on Sephadex G-50 (Fig. 9) and polyacrylamide gel electrophoresis (Fig. 10). These incubations were done with slices of whole pituitaries, which explains the low specific activity of the material obtained. The addition of a carrier (50 gm of fresh bovine pituitaries) is essential to increase extraction yields. However, there are indications from immunohistochemical investigations that β-LPH and β-MSH are more concentrated in the pars intermedia. Preliminary experi-

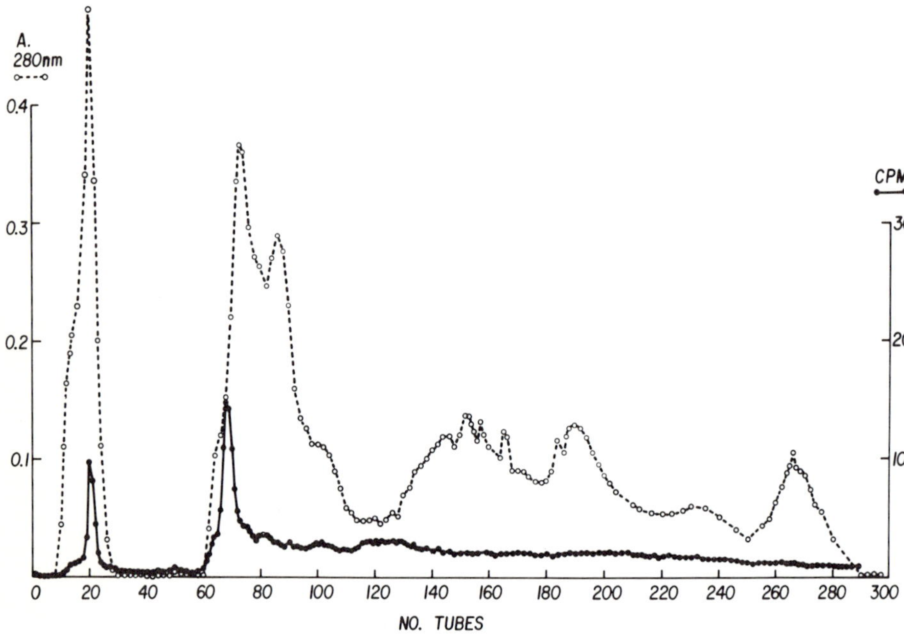

FIG. 8. CM cellulose chromatography of a fraction D. The column was 40 × 1 cm. A continuous gradient was started at tube 20 by the addition of 0.01 *M* NH_4Ac buffer, pH 6.7, to a 250-ml mixing chamber containing 0.01 *M* buffer pH 4.6. At tube 160, a 0.2 *M* NH_4Ac solution was used to increase the gradient. Fractions of 2 ml were collected at a rate of 1 ml/minute.

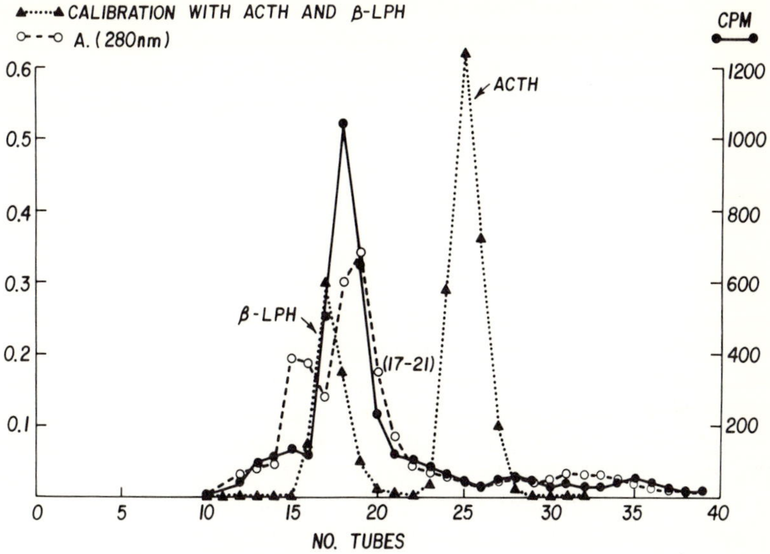

FIG. 9. Sephadex G-50 column chromatography (40 × 1 cm) of tubes 61–80 (Fig. 8) in 0.01 *M* NH_4OAc buffer, pH 4.6. Pure β-LPH and ACTH were used to calibrate the column.

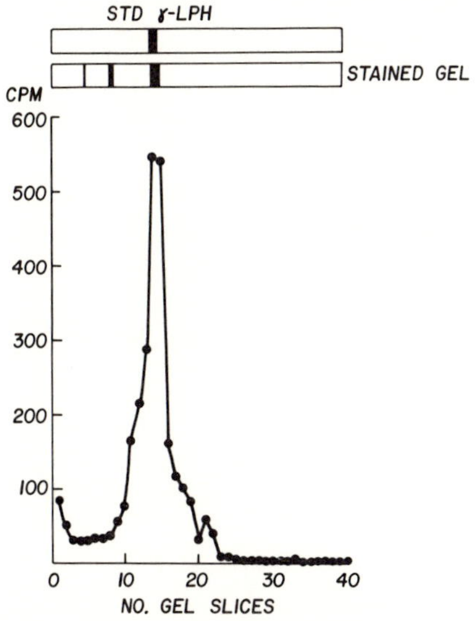

FIG. 10. Polyacrylamide gel electrophoresis at pH 4.5 (β-alanine buffer 0.35 *M*) of a pure preparation of γ-LPH and of two samples of peaks 17–21 (Fig. 9). One gel was stained, and the other was cut into 1-mm slices for radioactivity determination.

ments with cells isolated from the pars intermedia showed that these cells from bovine pituitaries are very unstable in incubation media.

The biosynthesis of γ-LPH in whole pituitaries is weak compared with that of the other pituitary hormones. This biosynthetic pathway needs to be stimulated if we are to follow, in a single experiment, the transformation of β-LPH into γ-LPH and hence (presumably) into β-MSH.

VI. Pituitary Cells Producing β-LPH

Many authors have studied by immunofluorescence and by peroxidase-conjugated antibody techniques the localization of pituitary cells containing β-LPH. Dessy *et al.* (1973) and Dubois and Gráf (1973) have found that most adrenocorticotroph cells in porcine pituitaries contains β-LPH and β-MSH. Dubois and Gráf (1973) and Moon *et al.* (1973) found that most adrenocorticotroph cells in porcine pituitaries contains studying normal human pituitary glands found that β-MSH and ACTH were contained in the same cells. Since, according to Scott and Lowry (1974) and Bloomfield *et al.* (1974), β-LPH is the main component of the β-MSH-β-LPH series in human glands, one can conclude that β-LPH will also be found in the same cells. Furth *et al.* (1975) confirmed these findings in human pituitaries and extend it to mice and rat pituitaries.

VII. Radioimmunoassay

The radioimmunoassay of ovine β-LPH was already described (Desranleau *et al.,* 1972; Desranleau and Chrétien, 1971). Recently, we have introduced with good results (M. Lis and M. Chrétien, unpublished results) the precipitation of bound β-LPH by means of polyethylene glycol as was proposed by Desbuquois and Aurbach (1971).

A. Specificity of the Assay

In the absence of β-LPH antiserum, the amount of ^{125}I-β-LPH precipitated by the second antibody was less than 4%. Rudman's peptide 7D6 and Trygastad's lipid-mobilizing factor (LMF) No. 6 showed a slight cross-reactivity ranging from 10 to 1000 ng and 10 to 20 ng, respectively. However, synthetic α-melanocyte-stimulating hormone (α-MSH), and ovine adrenocorticotropic hormone (ACTH) showed no cross-reaction with ovine β-LPH up to a dose of 1000 ng. Trygstad's LMF (s) No. 4 and No. 5 showed no cross-reaction with ovine β-LPH when tested up to 20 ng. Porcine β-LPH cross-reacted strongly with our sheep system. We attempted to neutralize this strong cross-reaction by adding 100 ng of porcine β-LPH to the incubation medium. The results showed that porcine β-LPH is immunologically closely related to ovine β-LPH. Two different human pituitary fractions isolated by M. Chrétien and G. Smith (unpublished results) had a slight, incomplete cross-reaction with sheep β-LPH. The specificity of the radioimmunoassay was also studied by demonstrating that the ^{125}I-β-LPH was almost completely immunoprecipitable (84%) in the presence of excess of specific antiserum and that it was not immunoprecipitable (4%) in the absence of specific antibody. As shown on the standard curve, the ^{125}I-β-LPH can be completely displaced from antibody by excess of unlabeled purified β-LPH.

Cyanogen bromide (CNBr) fragments (1–47 and 1–65) of ovine β-LPH reacted strongly with β-LPH antiserum. In fact, they had higher affinity to the antibodies than the complete molecule of ovine β-LPH. This suggests that some part of fragment 66–90 could inhibit the antigen–antibody reaction.

B. Measurement of a β-LPH-like Substance in Human Pituitary Gland and in Ovine and Human Serum

We were able to measure β-LPH in normal sheep serum. We used 200 ml of sheep serum dialyzed against distilled water (pH adjusted to 8.6 with 1.0 N NH_4OH) (at 4° C) and concentrated 5 times on a UM 2 membrane with an Amicon Diaflo ultrafilter. Sheep serum contained about 10 ng of β-LPH per milliliter. In saline extracts of one human pituitary gland removed surgically, we detected 1.70 μg equivalents of ovine β-LPH by the double antibody technique, and 1.56 with the method using dextran-coated charcoal.

However, in human serum, we were unable to detect β-LPH-like material. This could be due to poor cross-reactivity between the material isolated from human pituitaries and our anti-β-LPH antiserum, to the low sensitivity of the assay or to other factors. Various investigators have described the presence of nonspecific inhibitors such as γ-globulin or complement in undiluted serum or plasma used in the double-antibody radioimmunoassay for insulin and other protein hormones. Several methods have been proposed to overcome this nonspecific interference: addition of EDTA to the reaction mixture, dilution of the serum sample, and stepwise acetone extraction. These approaches were unsuccessful.

VIII. Biologic Activities of Lipotropins

A. Lipolytic and Melanophore-Stimulating Effects

Very little is known about the physiological effects of pituitary lipotropic hormones. All the components purified by different authors have *in vivo* and *in vitro* lipolytic effects. Ovine β- and γ-LPH and porcine and bovine β-LPH have also intrinsic melanophore-stimulating activity. This is not surprising because their structures contain a segment entirely identical with the β-MSH.

Table VI shows comparison of these two activities in β-MSH, ACTH, Rudman's peptides, and the different LPH's. It reveals that β-MSH (portion 41–58 of β-LPH) is 90–100 times more active than β-LPH and γ-LPH. As noted earlier, CNBr fragments (1–47, 48–91) have less than 10% β_s-LPH potency. But a synthetic fragment 48–91 is at least 6 times more active than the natural hormone (Yamashiro and Li, 1974). Thus, the addition of an hexapeptide (Ser-Gly-Pro-Tyr-Lys-Met) at the NH_2-terminus of residues 48–91 greatly increases the lipolytic activity.

It can be seen that, although peptide 7D7 is chemically different from β- and γ-LPH, it has an identical lipolytic activity in the rabbit, but it also has an hyperglycemic effect. Chrétien *et al.* (1970), however, have demonstrated that ovine β-LPH does not cause any change in plasma glucose levels.

Chrétien *et al.* (1970) have shown that highly purified ovine β-LPH has an intrinsic *in vivo* lipolytic activity in the rabbit. Their results are comparable with those of Tamasi *et al.* (1969) with porcine β-LPH. Plasma free

TABLE VI—Biologic Activities of Lipolytic Hormones

Hormones	MSH activity *in vitro* (U/g)	Lipolytic activity *in vitro* (MED)	
		Rabbit adipose tissue (μg)	Rat adipose tissue (μg)
Sheep γ-LPH	1.6×10^7	0.01	Not active
Sheep β-LPH	2.0×10^7	0.008	0.124
Porcine β-LPH	2.5×10^7	0.010	Not tested
Bovine β-LPH	2.0×10^7	0.0094	Not tested
β-MSH	1.2×10^9	0.0006	Not active
Human LPH (ours)	1.77×10^7	0.005	Not tested
Rudman's 7D7[a]	Not reported	0.01	Not active
Rudman's 7D6	Not reported	0.1	Not active
Acth	4×10^7	0.008	0.001

[a] Is also hyperglycemic and hypoaminoacidemic.

fatty acids (FFA) increase within 15 minutes and reach a peak 30–45 minutes after the injection.

B. Hypocalcemic Effect

Chrétien *et al.* (1970) also studied the effects of pure β-LPH on some other plasma constituents. They found that β-LPH did not affect plasma cholesterol, triglycerides, glucose, and magnesium but produced a significant decrease in plasma calcium, which reached a minimum between 120 and 180 minutes after iv administration.

Four rabbits were injected iv with 0.2 mg of β-LPH 2 weeks following thyroidectomy and FFA and calcium were again measured. Thyroidectomy affected slightly the lipolytic response but abolished the hypocalcemic effect. Treatment of thyroidectomized rabbits with triiodothyronine partly restored the hypocalcemic effect of β-LPH.

Our findings on the calcium lowering effect of pure ovine β-LPH confirm the results of others (Natelson *et al.,* 1963; Friesen, 1964; Trygstad, 1967) who used semipurified preparations of similar substances. The mechanism of action of β-LPH on calcium metabolism is not known. Akgun and Rudman (1969) reported that ACTH favors the entry of calcium into adipose tissue. Yanagi *et al.* (1969) showed the same with radioactive calcium. Our studies revealed that *in vivo* lipolysis is not necessarily accompanied by hypocalcemia and that the thyroid gland is necessary for β-LPH to produce its full hypocalcemic effect. Avioli *et al.* (1969) and Care *et al.* (1969) have recently reported that glucagon, also a lipolytic and hypocalcemic agent, stimulates calcitonin secretion. One, thus, could speculate if β-LPH acts on calcitonin-secreting cells indirectly by stimulating the release of glucagon. However, the absence of hyperglycemia following the injection of β-LPH makes this hypothesis unlikely. Moreover, Williams *et al.* (1969) showed that glucagon and calcitonin, in the rat, cause hypocalcemia by different mechanisms. It is interesting to note that sheep β-LPH does not cause any change in plasma magnesium level, in contrast to ACTH which, according to Akgun *et al.* (1969) causes an elevation of plasma magnesium. These last authors also found an increase in plasma triglycerides following injections of ACTH. This was not seen in our experiments, but we measured plasma triglycerides only during the first 4 hours following the injection.

C. Effect on Lipogenesis

Studies performed by Gattereau *et al.* (1970) indicate that β-LPH incubated with rat epididymal fat pads in Krebs–Ringer bicarbonate buffer stimulates the oxidation of glucose and its incorporation into fatty acids.

D. Effect on Coagulation

During *in vivo* experiments with β-LPH in rabbits, we noticed that samples of blood were coagulating more rapidly when lipolysis was at its maximum. Preliminary data (Chrétien *et al.,* 1971) reveal that β-LPH causes a significant decrease in coagulation time. This decrease was biphasic with peaks at 60 and 100 minutes, which were coincidental with the lipolysis and the hypocalcemia. Moreover, we were able to demonstrate that fibrinogen was concomitantly activated and that platelets adhesiveness was also increased. Plasma recalcification time was not affected.

E. Effect of Chemical Modifications on Biologic Activities

The modification of the tryptophan residue of ACTH by *o*-nitrophenyl sulfenyl chloride (NSP-ACTH) produced changes in lipolytic activity (Ramachandran and Lee, 1970). The same modifications of ovine β-LPH (NPS-β-LPH) changed the lipolytic activity of β-LPH as well. Both NPS-ACTH and NPS-β-LPH lost their lipolytic activity on rat fat preparations while retaining its lipolytic effect on rabbit fat preparations. In rat fat cells incubated *in vitro,* NPS-β-LPH behaved essentially the same way as NPS-ACTH. This seems to indicate that the receptors for β-LPH in fat tissue are related, if not identical, to those of ACTH and β-MSH (M. Lis and M. Chrétien, unpublished observations).

Using modification of the carboxyl groups with glycine methyl ester and taurine, Gilardeau *et al*. (1974) showed that LPH partially loses its lipolytic activity. When applied to the ACTH molecule, it was interesting to note that it loses its adrenocorticotropic activity, while the lipolytic activity in rabbit fat tissue *in vitro* is preserved.

IX. Mechanism of Action of β-LPH at the Cellular Level

Maximal and semimaximal doses of β-LPH were used to verify the stimulating activity on adenylate cyclase in adipose tissue. Lis *et al*. (1973) found in rats that β-LPH, like ACTH in comparable doses, produces a rapid accumulation of cyclic adenosine monophosphate (cAMP), reaching a maximum at about the tenth minute and returning to the baseline level after 40 minutes (Fig. 11). In the rabbit, on the other hand, there is a continuous increase up to 40 minutes. We had already observed, in fact, that the peak lipolytic response in the isolated rabbit cell is generally obtained after 2 hours, whereas it occurs after 1 hour in the rat cell (Chrétien *et al.,* 1970).

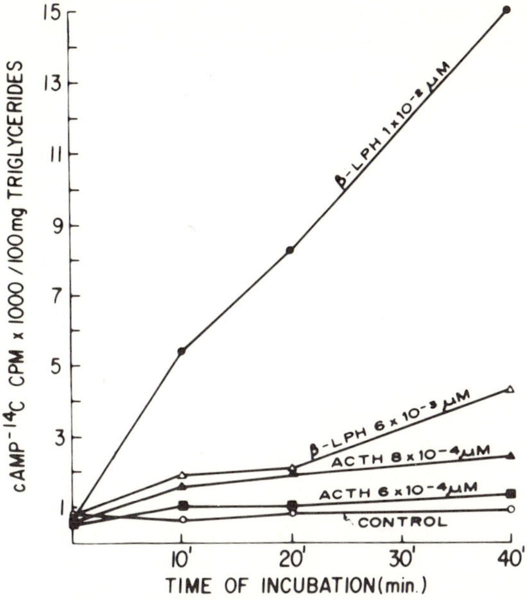

FIG. 11. Stimulation of adenylate cyclase by β-LPH and by ACTH in the rabbit. Adenylate cyclase activity is measured by the production of ^{14}C-cyclic AMP in isolated cells preincubated with ^{14}C-adenine. Doses of β-LPH and ACTH giving a lipolytic response 50% that of maximum stimulation were employed.

X. Physicochemical Studies of Sheep β-LPH

The near-ultraviolet circular dichroism spectra of sheep β-lipotropic hormone were recorded under different conditions of pH, temperature, and salt concentration (St-Pierre *et al.,* 1975). Results revealed that β-LPH is very stable in strong basic and acidic conditions, and temperatures up to 50° do not seem to affect its conformation. However, increasing NaCl concentration in the solution brings about a conformation transition of the chain, interpreted as an increase in the helical content. Table VII shows the predicted assignments attributed to the 91 amino acids, and Table VIII shows the comparisons between the theoretical structure and the actual CD results.

XI. Summary and Conclusions

Of all pituitary lipolytic peptides, sheep β-LPH has been the best studied. Not only do we know its chemical nature, but we understand better its biosynthesis, its biologic activities and its mechanism of action

TABLE VII—Predicted Helical, β-Sheet, and Turn Regions of β-LPH Including Conformational Parameters $P\alpha$, $P\beta$, P_t, and p_t

Fragment	Predicted structure	$P\alpha$	$P\beta$	P_t	$p_t \times 10^4$
*1–2	Coil	1.43	0.74	0.48	—
3–6	Turn	0.92	0.79	1.03	0.51
*7–9	Coil	1.35	0.90	0.51	—
10–13	Turn	0.84	0.83	1.21	0.61
14–27	Helical	1.35	0.69	—	—
28–32	Beta	1.01	1.18	—	—
33–39	Helical	1.34	0.63	—	—
40–42	Turn	—	—	1.38	0.57
43–46	Turn	—	—	1.37	2.27
47–52	Helical	1.17	1.00	0.77	—
*53–54	Coil	0.66	0.77	1.62	—
55–58	Turn	—	—	1.34	0.79
59–62	Turn	—	—	1.24	0.95
63–66	Beta	0.92	1.24	1.02	—
67–70	Coil	1.05	0.5	1.14	0.22
71–79	Beta	1.04	1.15	—	—
80–87	Coil	1.08	0.98	—	—
88–91	Turn	—	—	1.07	0.67

P_t is referred to as the turn parameter and p_t is the relative probability that a tetrapeptide will form a β-turn.

p_t = fi*fi-1*fi-2*fi-3 where the f's are, in that order, the frequency of occurrence for a certain residue at the first, second, third, and fourth position of a β-turn.

in whole animals and at the cellular level. It has lipolytic as well as melanophore-stimulating activity; it is a strong hypocalcemic agent in rabbits, and this is probably due in part to a marked shift of calcium in

TABLE VIII—Secondary Structure of β-LPH Predicted from the Primary Structure (Method of Chou and Fasman) Compared with Secondary Structure Assessed by CD (Method of Chen and Al)

	Helix	Beta (%)	Turn	Coil
Prediction	29.6	19.8	29.7	20.9
CD[a]	11.5	16.1		72.4
CD[b]	19.9	19.4		60.7

[a] 37°C, pH 7.40, 0 *M* NaCl.
[b] 37°C, pH 7.40, 5 *M* NaCl.

adipose cells during acute lipolysis; it causes a state of blood hypercoagu-bility secondary to increase in platelets adhesiveness. It stimulates cyclic AMP production, as does other lipolytic agents. The most important aspect of the biology of β-LPH is the fact that it is most likely the biologic precursor of β-MSH. This model of biosynthesis was proposed at the same time as Steiner's proinsulin. The discovery of γ-LPH by Chrétien and Li (1967a,b) was unique in that it was the first intermediate compound to be identified between a precursor and its active molecule. We now have been able to demonstrate that there is active biosynthesis of β-LPH and γ-LPH in fresh pituitaries, but this is a slow process, which has prevented us so far from showing directly their transformation into β-MSH.

XII. Addendum

Since Hughes *et al.* (1975) discovered met-enkephalin, a substance which is made up of residues 61–65 of β-LPH, other endogenous opiate substances, mainly β-endorphin (made of residues 61–91 of β-LPH) have been isolated (Li and Chung, 1976; Bradbury *et al.*, 1976; Guillemin *et al.*, 1976; Chrétian *et al.*, 1976).

The pituitary glands from at least 4 species contain β-LPH and β-endorphin (Li and Chung, 1976; Bradbury *et al.*, 1976; Guillemin *et al.*, 1976; Chrétian *et al.*, 1976). We have shown that in slices of whole pituitaries, β-LPH is actively biosynthesized and transformed into γ-LPH, thus releasing the C-terminus portion 61–91, which is now known as β-endorphin. Newly radioactive biosynthesized β-endorphin has been clearly and definitely identified. The release of β-MSH and possibly of β-endorphin could well be under the control of corticotropin releasing hormone.

The intermediate lobe of the pituitary seems to be the tissue which contains most of β-LPH and β-endorphin, although these are also present in the anterior lobe. We have recently demonstrated the presence of β-endorphin in both human and sheep glands and the structure is identical to the C-fragment 61–91 of their respective β-LPH (Chrétien *et al.*, 1976; Dragon *et al.*, 1977; Seidah *et al.*, 1977).

Until somebody shows that β-LPH and β-endorphin are actively biosynthesized in other tissues, one can only assume that the pituitary gland is the primary source of the endogenous opiate substance(s) and that β-LPH is its or their biological precursor.

The major conclusion of our most recent studies on the biosynthesis of β-LPH and its related peptides have led us to the first *in vitro* biosynthesis of an endogenous morphinelike substance (Crine *et al.*, 1977a,b). This constitutes a major step in the comprehension of this exciting new field.

Acknowledgment

Work published in this review was supported by Medical Research Council of Canada grants, the Quebec Heart Foundation, the National Cancer Institute of Canada and "le Ministère de l'Education du Québec".

The authors wish to thank Mrs. D. Marcil for her excellent secretarial assistance.

References

Abdurankhmanov, G. A., and Lipovetzky, B. M. (1966). *Vopr. Med. Khim.* **12,** 355.

Akgun, S., and Rudman, D. (1969). *Endocrinology* **84,** 926.

Akgun, S., Rudman, D., and Wertheim, A. R. (1969). *Endocrinology* **84,** 347.

Anselmino, K. J., and Hoffmann, F. (1931). *Klin. Wochenschr.* **10,** 2380.

Astwood, E. B., Barrett, R. J., and Friesen, H. (1961). *Proc. Natl. Acad. Sci. U. S. A.* **47,** 1525.

Avioli, L. V., Birge, S. J., Scott, S., and Shieber, W. (1969). *Gastroenterology* **57,** 468.

Bertagna, S., Lis, M., Gilardeau, C., and Chrétien. M. (1974). *Can. J. Biochem.* **52,** 349.

Best, C. H., and Campbell, J. (1936). *J. Physiol. (London)* **86,** 190.

Birk, Y., and Li, C. H. (1964). *J. Biol. Chem.* **239,** 1048.

Bloomfield, G. A., Scott, A. P., Lowry, P. G., Gilkes, J. J. H., and Rees, L. H. (1974). *Nature (London)* **252,** 492.

Bradbury, A. F., Smyth, D. G., and Snell, C. R. (1976). *Biochem. Biophys. Res. Commun.* **69,** 950–956.

Burns, T. S., Hales, C. N., and Hartree, A. S. (1967). *J. Endocrinol.* **39,** 213.

Care, A. D., Bates, R. F. L., and Gitelman, H. J. (1969). *J. Endocrinol.* **43,** 55.

Chance, R. E., Ellis, R. M., and Bromer, W. W. (1968). *Science* **161,** 165.

Chrétien, M. (1968). *Union Med. Can.* **97,** 166.

Chrétien, M. (1973). *In* "Peptide Hormones" (S. A. Berson and R. S. Yalow, eds.), Vol. 2A, p. 617. North-Holland Publ., Amsterdam.

Chrétien, M., and Gilardeau, C. (1969). *Proc. Can. Fed. Biol. Soc.* **12,** 63.

Chrétien, M., and Gilardeau, C. (1970). *Can. J. Biochem.* **48,** 511.

Chrétien, M., and Li, C. H. (1967a). *Can. J. Biochem.* **45,** 1163.

Chrétien, M., and Li, C. H. (1967b). *Can. Med. Assoc. J.* **96,** 343.

Chrétien, M., Davignon, J., Lis, M., Chari, P. V., Aubry, F., and Gilardeau, C. (1970). *Can. J. Physiol. Pharmacol.* **48,** 762.

Chrétien, M., Dufault, C., Gratton, J., and Gilardeau, C. (1971). *Horm. Metab. Res.* **3,** 355.

Chrétien, M., Gilardeau, C., Lis, M., and Benjannet, S. (1975). *Can. J. Biochem.* (submitted for publication).

Chrétien, M., Benjannet, S., Dragon, N., Seidah, N. G., and Lis, M. (1976). *Biochem. Biophys. Res. Commun.* **72,** 472–478.

Cohn, D. V., MacGregor, R. R., Chu, L. L. H., Kimmel, J. R., and Hamilton, J. W. (1972). *Proc. Natl. Acad. Sci. U. S. A.* **69,** 1521.

Crine, P., Benjannet, S., Seidah, N. G., Lis, M., and Chrétien, M. (1977a). *Proc. Natl. Acad. Sci. U. S. A.* **74,** 1403–1406.

Crine, P., Benjannet, S., Seidah, N. G., Lis, M., and Chrétien, M. (1977b). (submitted for publication).

Cseh, G., Gráf, L., and Goth, E. (1968). *FEBS Lett.* **2,** 42.

Cseh, G., Barat, E., Patthy, A., and Gráf, L. (1972). *FEBS Lett.* **21,** 344.

Desbuquois, B., Aurbach, G. D. (1971). *J. Clin. Endocrinol. Metab.* **33,** 732.

Desranleau, R., and Chrétien, M. (1971). *Union Med. Can.* **100,** 782.

Desranleau, R., Gilardeau, C., and Chrétien, M. (1972). *Endocrinology* **91,** 1004.

Dessy, C., Herlant, M., and Chrétien, M. (1973). *C.R. Hebd. Seances Acad. Sci.* **276,** 335.

Dragon, N., Seidah, N. G., Lis, M., Routhier, R., and Chrétien, M. (1977). *Can. J. Biochem.* (in press).

Dubois, M. P., and Gráf, L. (1973). *Horm. Metab. Res.* **5,** 229.

Freinkel, N. (1961). *J. Clin. Invest.* **40,** 476.

Friesen, H. (1964). *Endocrinology* **75,** 692.

Furth, J., Chrétien, M., Moy, P., and Grauman, J. (1975). *Arch. Pathol.* **99,** 572.

Gattereau, A., Chrétien, M., and Bielmann, P. (1970). *Horm. Metab. Res.* **2,** 330.

Gilardeau, C., and Chrétien, M. (1970a). *Can. J. Biochem.* **48,** 1017.

Gilardeau, C., and Chrétien, M. (1970b). *Proc. Can. Fed. Biol. Soc.* **13,** 100.

Gilardeau, C., and Chrétien, M. (1972). *In* "Chemistry and Biology of Peptides" (J. Meinenhofer, ed.), p. 609. Ann Arbor Sci. Publ., Ann Arbor, Michigan.

Gilardeau, C., Chrétien, M., and Lis, M. (1974). *Can. J. Physiol. Pharmacol.* **52,** 723.

Goth, E., Cseh, G., Fovenzi, J., and Gráf, L. (1969). *Kiserl. Orvostud.* **21,** 277.

Gráf, L., and Cseh, G. (1968). *Acta Biochim. Biophys. Acad. Sci. Hung.* **3,** 175.

Gráf, L., Cseh, G., and Schweizer, J. M. (1969). *Biochim. Biophys. Acta* **175,** 444.

Gráf, L., Barat, E., Cseh, G., and Sajgo, M. (1971). *Biochim. Biophys. Acta* **229,** 276.

Gráf, L., Barat, E., Patthy, A., and Cseh, G. (1974). *Arch. Biochem. Biophys.* **161,** 211.

Guillemin, R., Ling, N., and Burgus, R. (1976). *C.R. Acad. Sci. Ser. D (Paris)* **282,** 783.

Habener, J. F., Kemper, B., Potts, J. T., Jr., and Rich, A. (1972). *Science* **178,** 630.

Habener, J. F., Kemper, B., Potts, J. T., and Rich, A. (1973). *Endocrinology* **92,** 219.

Hoffmann, K., and Katsoyannis, P. G. (1963). *Proteins, 2nd Ed.* **1,** 138.

Hollenberg, M. D., and Hope, D. B. (1968). *Biochem. J.* **106,** 557.

Hughes, J., Smith, T. W., Kosterlitz, H. W., Fothergill, L. A., Morgan, B. A., and Morris, H. R. (1975). *Nature (London)* **258,** 577–579.

Kemper, B., Habener, J. F., Potts, J. T., and Rich, A. (1972). *Proc. Natl. Acad. Sci. U. S. A.* **69,** 643.

Kemper, B., Habener, J. F., Mulligan, R. C., Potts, J. T., and Rich, A. (1974). *Proc. Natl. Acad. Sci. U. S. A.* **71,** 3731.

Leites, S. M., and Davtyan, N. K. (1963). *Byull. Eksp. Biol. Med.* **55,** 60.

Leites, S. M., and Davtyan, N. K. (1965a). *Vopr. Med. Khim.* **11,** 49.

Leites, S. M., and Davtyan, N. K. (1965b). *Byull. Eksp. Biol. Med.* **59,** 55.

Li, C. H. (1964). *Nature (London)* **201,** 924.

Li, C. H., and Chung, D. (1976). *Proc. Natl. Acad. Sci. U. S. A.* **73,** 1145–1148.

Li, C. H., Barnafi, L., Chrétien, M., and Chung, D. (1965). *Nature (London)* **208,** 1093.

Li, C. H., Barnafi, L., Chrétien, M., and Chung, D. (1966). *Proc. Pan-Am. Congr. Endocrinol., 6th 1965* Excerpta Med. Found. Int. Congr. Ser. No. 112, p. 349.

Lis, M., Gilardeau, C., and Chrétien, M. (1972). *Proc. Soc. Exp. Biol. Med.* **139,** 680.

Lis, M., Gilardeau, C., and Chrétien, M. (1973). *Comp. Biochem. Physiol. B* **46,** 661.

Lohmar, P., and Li, C. H. (1967). *Biochim. Biophys. Acta* **147,** 381.

Moon, H. D., Li, C. H., and Jennings, B. M. (1973). *Anat. Rec.* **175,** 529.

Natelson, S., Pincus, J. B., and Rannazzisi, G. (1963). *Clin. Chem.* **9,** 31.

Noe, B. D., and Bauer, G. E. (1971). *Endocrinology* **89,** 642.

Noe, B. D., and Bauer, G. E. (1973). *Proc. Soc. Exp. Biol. Med.* **142,** 210.

Phifer, R. F., Orth, D. N., and Spicer, S. S. (1974). *J. Clin. Endocrinol. Metab.* **39,** 684.

Preddie, E. C., and Saffran, M. (1965). *J. Biol. Chem.* **240,** 4189.

Raben, M. S., Landolt, R., Smith, F. A., Hoffmann, K., and Yajima, H. (1961). *Nature (London)* **189,** 681.

Ramachandran, J., and Lee, N. M. (1970). *Biochem. Biophys. Res. Commun.* **38,** 507.

Rauch, R., Hollenberg, M. D., and Hope, D. B. (1969). *Biochem. J.* **115,** 473.

Rigopoulou, D., Valverde, I., Marco, J., Faloona, G. R., and Unger, R. H. (1970). *J. Biol. Chem.* **245,** 496.

Rishka, F. Y., and Khokhlov, A. S. (1965). *Biokhymia* **30,** 1277.

Rudman, D., and Seidman, F. (1958). *Proc. Soc. Exp. Biol. Med.* **99,** 146.

Rudman, D., Brown, S. J., and Malkin, M. F. (1963). *Endocrinology* **72,** 527.

Rudman, D., Del Rio, A. E., Gardia, L. A., Barnette, J., Howard, C. H., Walker, W., and Moore, G. (1970). *Biochemistry* **9,** 99.

St-Pierre, S., Gilardeau, C., and Chrétien, M. (1976). *Can. J. Biochem.* **54,** 992.

Schleyer, M., Straub, K., and Pfeiffer, E. F. (1969a). *Horm. Metab. Res.* **1,** 201.

Schleyer, M., Straub, K., Faulhaber, J. D., and Pfeiffer, E. F. (1969b). *Horm. Metab. Res.* **1,** 286.

Schwandt, P., Werner, S., and Karl, H. J. (1968). *Z. Gesamte Exp. Med.* **148,** 164.

Schwandt, P., Weisweiler, P., and Eicher, R. (1969). *Klin. Wochenschr.* **47,** 1174.

Scott, A. P., and Lowry, P. J. (1974). *Biochem. J.* **139,** 593.

Seidah, N. G., Dragon, N., Benjannet, S., Routhier, R., and Chrétien, M. (1977). *Biochem. Biophys. Res. Commun.* **74,** 1528–1535.

Smith, G. (1973). "A New Lipolytic-Melanotropic Peptide from Human Pituitary." McGill University, Montreal.

Smith, G., Gilardeau, C., Lis, M., and Chrétien, M. (1976). *Rev. Can. Biol.* **35,** 51.

Steiner, D. F., Cunningham, D., Spiegelman, L., and Aten, B. (1967). *Science* **157,** 967.

Steiner, D. F., Hallund, O., Rubenstein, A., Cho, S., and Bayliss, C. (1968). *Diabetes* **17,** 725.

Tager, H. S., and Steiner, D. F. (1973). *Proc. Natl. Acad. Sci. U. S. A.* **70,** 2321.

Tamasi, G., Cseh, G., and Gráf, L. (1969). *Experientia* **25,** 360.

Tanaka, A., Pickering, B. T., and Li, C. H. (1962). *Arch. Biochem. Biophys.* **99,** 294.

Trygstad, O. (1965). *Acta Endocrinol. (Copenhagen), Suppl.* **100,** 144.

Trygstad, O. (1967). *Acta Endocrinol. (Copenhagen)* **56,** 626.

Trygstad, O. (1968). *Acta Endocrinol. (Copenhagen)* **57,** 81.

Trygstad, O., and Foss, I. (1967). *Acta Endocrinol. (Copenhagen)* **56,** 649.

White, J. E., and Engel, F. L. (1958). *Proc. Soc. Exp. Biol. Med.* **99,** 375.

Williams, G. A., Bowser, E. N., and Henderson, W. J. (1969). *Endocrinology* **85,** 537.

Wuu, T. C., and Saffran, M. (1969). *J. Biol. Chem.* **244,** 482.

Yamashiro, D., and Li, C. H. (1974). *Proc. Natl. Acad. Sci. U.S.A.* **71,** 4945.

Yanagi, I., Okuda, H., and Fujii, S. (1969). *J. Biochem. (Tokyo)* **66,** 99.

Yip, C. C. (1968). *Arch. Biochem. Biophys.* **127,** 741.

Yudaev, N. A., and Pankov, Y. A. (1970). *Probl. Endocrinol.* **16,** 49.

4

The Neurophysins

B. T. PICKERING AND C. W. JONES

I. The Discovery of the Neurophysins

During the first few years of this century, extracts of the posterior pituitary gland were found to be endowed with a number of biologic activities. Besides raising the blood pressure of mammals (Oliver and Schafer, 1895), they were vasodepressor in birds (Paton and Watson, 1912), antidiuretic in man (von den Velden, 1913; Farini, 1913), promoted milk flow in lactating goats (Ott and Scott, 1910), and caused contraction of the guinea pig uterus—the so-called oxytocic effect (Dale, 1906, 1909). There was considerable discussion as to whether there was present in the posterior pituitary gland a single molecule endowed with all of these biologic activities or a number of biologically active compounds. This controversy was still not resolved when Dudley (1919, 1923) showed that a fraction rich in antidiuretic and pressor activities could be separated from one enriched in oxytocic and avian vasodepressor properties, nor when Kamm *et al*. (1928) extended Dudley's techniques to achieve such separations readily enough for commercial use, since it was held (Abel, 1924, 1930) that separation of the activities could have been brought about by degradation of the parent hormone.

In defense of the "unitary" hypothesis, several workers (MacArthur, 1931; Rosenfield, 1940) reported evidence for the presence of a large polypeptide having both oxytocic and vasopressor activities, and, in 1942, van Dyke and his colleagues showed that the addition of sodium chloride to acid extracts of bovine neurohypophyses resulted in precipitation of a protein having all of the biologic actions of posterior pituitary extracts in the proportions found in the gland. This "van Dyke protein" had a molecular weight (MW) of about 30,000 and was rich in cystine (Block and van Dyke, 1952).

The nature of the van Dyke protein was studied by Fromageot and his colleagues (see Acher and Fromageot, 1957), and, in 1955, Acher *et al.* isolated the protein part of the complex and coined the name neurophysine. The French workers showed that the van Dyke protein was a noncovalently linked complex, which could be reconstituted by mixing neurophysin, oxytocin, and vasopressin and precipitating with sodium chloride, and we now know that this complex is held together by ionic bonds involving the α-amino group of the hormones (Ginsburg and Ireland, 1963, 1964; Stouffer *et al.,* 1963).

In 1957, Acher and Fromageot concluded their paper thus: "Further investigations are necessary to determine whether the complex formed by vasopressin, oxytocin and inert protein is an artifact or whether it has biological significance." As this chapter will show, many "further investigations" have been made and, although still more are necessary, we can now be confident that the complex, and more especially the "inert protein," does have biologic significance, even if we are not all agreed what this significance is. Such is the current interest in neurophysin that the New York Academy of Sciences organized a 3-day symposium devoted entirely to it, and the reader is directed to the proceedings of this meeting (Walter, 1975), as well as to the reviews of Breslow (1974), Hope and Pickup (1974), and Acher (1976) for more detailed information about the studies discussed in this chapter.

II. Properties of the Neurophysins

Although in the sections to follow, the structural and biochemical features of the individual neurophysins will be discussed in some detail, it is perhaps appropriate to make some general comments on their properties. Neurophysin is known particularly as a sulfur-rich protein but the first attempts at determination of the amino acid composition (of the van Dyke protein) showed there to be a great abundance of glutamic acid, glycine, and proline residues, as well as a high proportion of cystine (Block and van Dyke, 1952). The presence of a large number of acidic residues endows the molecule (p*I* 4.5–5.0) with a high mobility in starch gel or polyacrylamide gel electrophoresis systems and has proved useful for the "identification" of putative neurophysins in glands from several species.

By definition, neurophysins form ionic complexes with the nonapeptide neurohypophyseal hormones, and, although the pH optimum for such complex formation is pH 5.8, they can be readily salted out at pH 3.9. Neurophysin itself is soluble in dilute 10% (v/v) NaCl at pH 3.9, but the addition of hormone leads to the precipitation of a protein–hormone complex (Stouffer *et al.*, 1963) that is insoluble enough to withstand dialysis and, thus, providing a useful intermediate in the purification of neurohypophyseal hormones (Acher *et al.*, 1958). A second, curious solubility property of the neurophysins and their hormone complexes, which has been useful in their isolation, is that they will dissolve in high concentrations (60–70%) of alcohol (MacArthur, 1931; Albers and Brightman, 1959). This property underlies the ability of relatively high concentrations of ethanol or acetone to extract porcine neurophysin during percolation of porcine pituitary glands (Friesen and Astwood, 1967; Wuu and Saffran, 1969a,b; Cheng and Friesen, 1971a). Martin *et al.* (1972) took advantage of this high solubility in their radioimmunoassay for bovine neurophysin. Addition of ethanol to a final concentration of 60% precipitates antibody-bound neurophysin, leaving the unbound protein in solution and, thus, allows the required separation of bound and free to be readily obtained.

Neurophysins also have unusual spectral properties (Fig. 1), since ϵ260 is greater than ϵ280. This property is also of use during purification, since a peak emerging from a chromatographic column can be tentatively identified as a neurophysinlike protein if its E_{280}/E_{260} ratio is about 0.8 (Hollenberg and Hope, 1967).

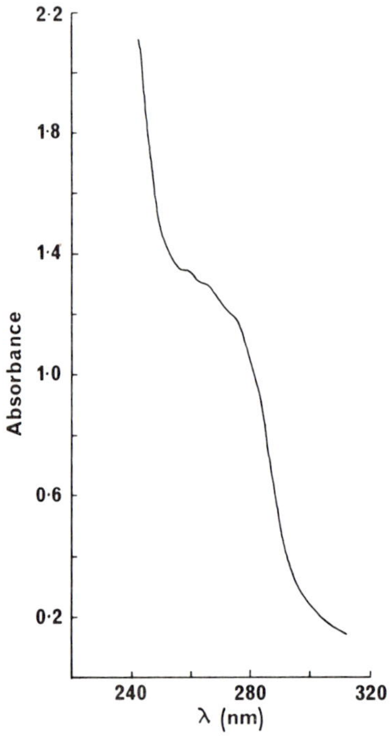

FIG. 1. Spectrum of bovine neurophysin II. A solution of 5 mg/ml in 0.1 *M* formic acid was examined in a cuvette of 1-cm light path.

III. Isolation and Composition of Neurophysins

The first attempts at characterizing neurophysin came before it had been so named and while its relationship to the hormones was still not understood. Van Dyke and co-workers (van Dyke *et al.*, 1942) were able to precipitate the protein–hormone complex from bovine neural lobe extracts using a salting out procedure. This crude preparation of active complex (now known to be neurophysin bound to hormone) was found to have a high sulfur content (4.9%) and appeared to be homogeneous as judged by constant solubility, ultracentrifugation, and electrophoresis. It had an MW of 24,000–30,000 from analytical and sedimentation data. Further studies on the amino acid composition of the protein by Block and van Dyke (1952) showed a high content of cystine and of dicarboxylic acids.

The next phase in the structural analysis of the neurophysins occurred in the late 1950's and involved the application of newly evolved separation techniques to the neurohypophyseal proteins. The extraction of neurophysin preparations from the acetone-dried powders of a number of species utilized the insolubility of the van Dyke protein–hormone complex at pH 4.0 in the presence of high sodium chloride concentrations. This protein–hormone complex was then dissociated either with trichloroacetic acid (TCA) (Chauvet *et al.,* 1960) or by gel filtration at low pH (Lindner *et al.,* 1959) to give the protein neurophysin(e) free from the hormones.

Early results suggested that the neurophysin prepared in this way was very heterogeneous. For example, Hollenberg and Hope (1967) used CM–Sephadex chromatography to separate a bovine preparation into seven components, each having a similar MW and amino acid composition. In a similar manner, Breslow and Abrash (1966) were able to resolve a bovine neurophysin preparation into 4 main components by DEAE–Sephadex chromatography and into 10 components by polyacrylamide gel electrophoresis (PAGE). When, however, Dean and Hope (1967) prepared neurosecretory granules from fresh bovine tissue, the granule lysate revealed only two major components on starch gel electrophoresis. Subsequently, Hope and collaborators, in studies which influenced the development of research into the chemistry of the neurophysins, were able to demonstrate that the heterogeneity previously found in neurophysin preparations was due, in part, to the extraction technique. It had been customary to extract posterior pituitaries with dilute acetic acid, which produces a pH in the extract close to the optimum for catheptic activity (Dean *et al.,* 1967). If bovine posterior pituitary acetone–powder is first extracted with 0.1 *N* HCl at low pH (<1.6), the catheptic activity is irreversibly destroyed, and starch gel electrophoresis of bovine neurophysin prepared at this low pH shows two major bands which are identical with those present in bovine neurosecretory granule lysates (Dean and Hope, 1968). Since this work was published, low pH has been universally employed to prepare posterior pituitary extracts from which a crude neurophysin–peptide complex could be precipitated by adding NaCl to a final concentration of 10%. A neurophysin concentrate has then been separated from the hormones and plasma protein contaminants by single or multiple gel filtration (Frankland *et al.,* 1966; Hollenberg and Hope, 1967; Breslow *et al.,* 1971). In general, ion-exchange chromatography has been used to fractionate this neurophysin concentrate into the individual neurophysin components. The recent search for the purest preparations of the neurophysins for sequence studies, and the realization that ion-exchange chromatography alone does not completely eliminate contaminating peptide material, has stimulated the search for more effective methods of purification, such as preparative PAGE (Walter *et al.*, 1971; Pliška *et al.*, 1972; Coy and Wuu, 1971, 1972; Capra *et al.*, 1974; Pickering *et al.*, 1975) and isoelectric focusing (Pliška *et al.*, 1972; Camier *et al.*, 1973).

A. Bovine

Starch gel electrophoresis of bovine neurosecretory granule lysates revealed two major and a number of minor components. The most prominent minor component designated c had an R_f between that of the two major ones, which on the basis of their relative electrophoretic mobilities had been designated bNpI and bNpII (Rauch *et al.*, 1969). Ion-exchange chromatography allowed the separation of the two major bovine neurophysins (Hollenberg and Hope, 1968) and the minor component c (Rauch *et al.*, 1969). All three proteins had a similar amino acid composition, being rich in cysteine, proline, glutamic acid, and glycine, but low in aromatic amino acid residues. End-group analysis gave a single NH_2-terminal amino acid, alanine, in each case. The other main differences were that NpI contained one residue/mole histidine but no methionine, whereas NpII and c had no histidine but contained one residue of methionine.

Confirmation of these findings came from Breslow *et al.* (1971) who purified two major neurophysins from acetone-dried, bovine, posterior pituitary material and obtained amino acid analyses almost identical to those of Rauch *et al.* (1969). Walter *et al.* (1971) reported an amino acid composition of bNpII which was identical to that obtained by Breslow *et al.* (1971), and went on to determine the sequence of the peptide. Table I shows the composition of the major and minor bovine peptides so far investigated. More recent studies have established the full sequence of bNpI with assignment of disulfide bridges (Fig. 2).

B. Porcine

Similarly two major and one minor neurophysins have been identified in the pig (Uttenthal and Hope, 1970; Friesen and Astwood, 1967; Cheng and Friesen, 1971a; Coy and Wuu, 1971). Uttenthal and Hope (1970) used

TABLE I—Amino Acid Composition of Bovine Neurophysins

Amino acid	Major components: Bovine NpI			Major components: Bovine NpII			Minor components bovine Npc
Lys	2[a]	2[b]	2[c]	2[a]	2[b,d]	2[e]	2[a]
His	1	1	1	0	0	0	0
Arg	4	4	4	7	7	7	5
Asp	7	7	7	5	5	5	6
Thr	2	2	2	2	2	2	2
Ser	6	5	6	6	6	6	7
Glu	10	11	9	14	14	13	14
Pro	9	9	9	8	8	8	9
Gly	15	14	14	16	16	15	16
Ala	9	9	8	6	6	6	7
½ Cys	12	14	14	14	14	14	14
Val	3	3	3	4	4	3/4	3
Met	0	0	0	1	1	1	1
Ile	2	2	2	2	2	2/3	2
Leu	6	6	7	6	6	6	7
Tyr	1	1	1	1	1	1	1
Phe	3	3	3	3	3	3	3

[a] Rauch *et al.* (1969).
[b] Breslow *et al.* (1971).
[c] Sequence of Schlesinger *et al.* (1977a).
[d] Walter *et al.* (1971).
[e] Sequence of Chauvet *et al.* (1976) and Wuu and Crumm (1976a).

a salt precipitation step in their purification procedure, while the other workers utilized a solvent–percolation method.

The percolation method of extraction, followed by ion-exchange chromatography, led to the isolation of two major peptides, II and III, and a minor component IV. Cheng and Friesen (1971a), on the basis of amino acid composition and electrophoretic mobility on starch gel electrophoresis, thought it likely that peptides II, III, and IV corresponded, respectively, with the porcine neurophysins designated I, II, and III by Uttenthal and Hope (1970), as well as to pNpII and pNpIII isolated by Coy and Wuu (1971) using preparative PAGE. The amino acid analyses for the analogous proteins were indeed very similar, and none of the porcine neurophysins isolated by any of these groups contained histidine. pNpI (peptide II) and pNpIII (peptide IV) contained one residue of methionine, while pNpII (peptide III) contained no methionine.

Wuu and Saffran (1969a,b) used a percolation method to isolate a

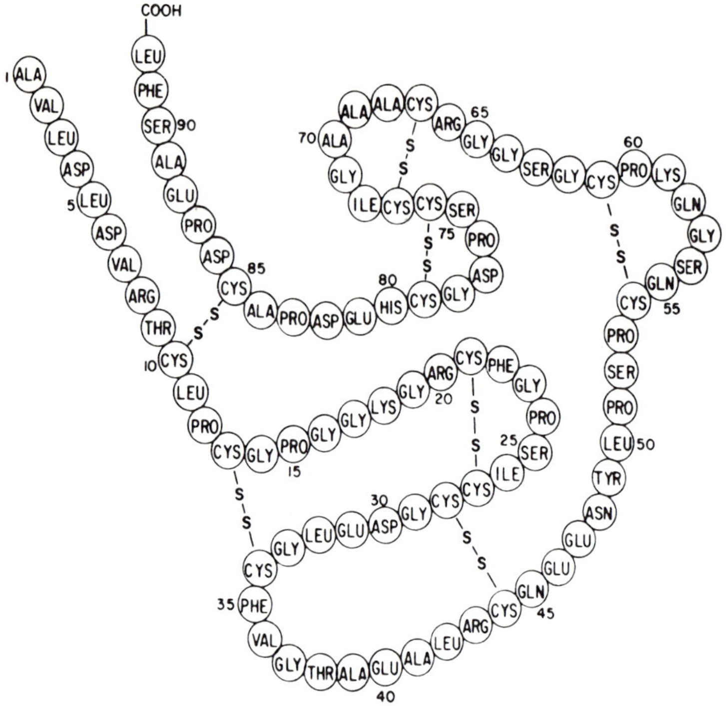

FIG. 2. The structure of bovine neurophysin I. (From North *et al.*, 1975, and Schlesinger *et al.*, 1977a.)

porcine polypeptide which bound lysine vasopressin. At the time, it was not classified as a neurophysin because of its "low" MW (about 9000). However, this was probably the first publication of the monomeric MW for a neurophysin, since the Wuu and Saffran peptide was almost certainly pNpI; its electrophoretic mobility was almost identical to that of peptide II (Cheng and Friesen, 1971a), and the amino acid analyses of the two preparations differed only by serine and proline. End-group analysis gave alanine as the NH_2-terminal amino acid and phenylalanine as the COOH-terminal residue.

Working from a slightly different standpoint, Rudman *et al.* (1970) isolated a lipolytic peptide from porcine pituitaries. This preparation had a composition similar to that of the porcine neurophysins, and its electrophoretic mobility on starch gel was identical to that of peptide II (Friesen, 1964) so it now appears that this peptide was pNpI. Thus, the pig, like the cow, has two major neurophysins and a minor component. Immunologic cross-reactivities suggested that bNpI and pNpII were immunologically related, as were bNpII and pNpI (Cheng and Friesen,

1971b). This finding fits in with the proposed biologic functions of these proteins (see below) and with structural similarities. Table II compares the composition of the porcine peptides isolated by a variety of investigators and techniques.

C. HUMAN

Recently, with the advent of radioimmunoassay and the possibility of a clinical application for neurophysin measurements, there has been a great deal of interest in the purification of neurophysins from human material.

Cheng and Friesen (1972) were the first to purify neurophysins from human sources and used, as starting material, the ethanol supernatant remaining after gonadotrophins had been extracted from whole acetone-dried pituitaries. Neurophysins were precipitated by acetone and then separated and purified by gel filtration and DEAE–cellulose chromatography. Two neurophysin components were isolated, each showing the

TABLE II—Amino Acid Composition of Porcine Neurophysins

Amino acid	Major components						Minor components		
	NpI			NpII			NpIII		
Lys	2[a]	2[b]	2[c]	4[d]	4[a]	4[c]	2[a]	2[c]	2[e]
His	0	0	0	0	0	0	0	0	0
Arg	5	5	5	7	6	6	6	6	7
Asp	5	5	5	7	12	9	5	5	5
Thr	2	2	2	2	3	2	2	2	2
Ser	8	7	6	6	9	6	7	6	7
Glu	13	13	13	20	15	11	12	11	13
Pro	7	7	7	8	14	10	6	6	7
Gly	14	14	14	8	20	14	13	13	14
Ala	7	7	7	6	12	9	8	7	8
$\frac{1}{2}$ Cys	12	14	13	13	18	16	12	12	14
Val	2	2	2	2	4	4	2	2	2
Met	1	1	1	2	0	0	1	1	1
Ile	2	2	2	2	3	2	2	2	2
Leu	7	7	7	8	9	7	7	7	7
Tyr	1	1	1	2	2	1	1	1	1
Phe	3	3	3	4	6	4	3	3	3

[a] Uttenthal and Hope (1970).
[b] Wuu *et al.* (1971).
[c] Cheng and Friesen (1971a).
[d] Rudman *et al.* (1970).
[e] Wuu and Crumm (1976b).

typical neurophysin UV absorption spectrum and having the same mobilities as the major bands detected during starch or polyacrylamide gel electrophoresis of homogenates of human posterior pituitary lobes. These were designated hNpI and hNpII by virtue of their respective mobilities in starch gel electrophoresis. In both starch gel and PAG electrophoresis, hNpI had a mobility very similar to pNpII, while hNpII had a mobility similar to those of pNpIII and bNpII (Fig. 3). The amino acid analyses of hNpI and hNpII were very similar, each containing one residue/mole of histidine. There was no methionine in hNpI, while hNpII contained a single residue. Both peptides bound LVP and the NH_2-terminal amino acid was shown to be alanine in each case.

Foss *et al.* (1973) used fresh-frozen pituitary glands, and an acetone precipitation step followed by DEAE–cellulose chromatography and purified a single protein with hormone-binding properties. This protein differed from that of Cheng and Friesen (1972) with regard to its content of arginine, proline, glycine, and alanine; a small content of methionine and

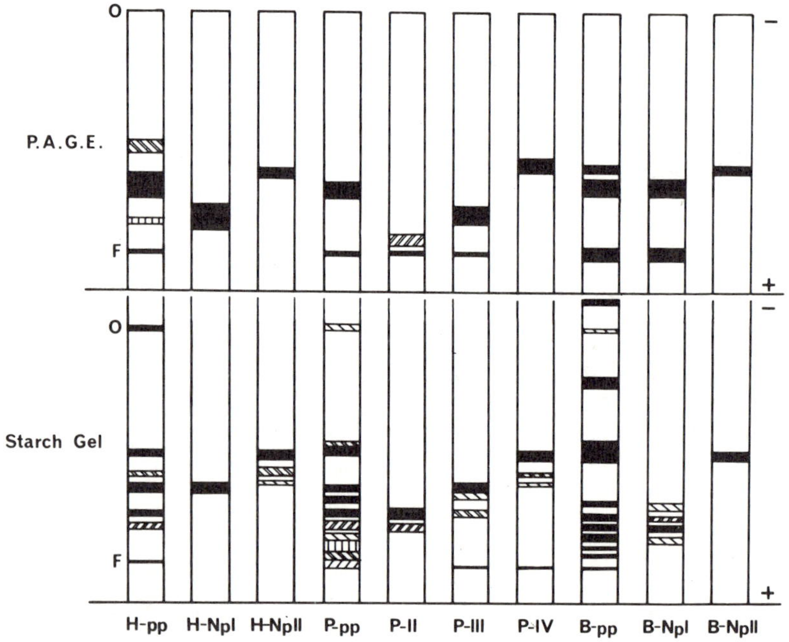

FIG. 3. Comparison of the electrophoretic mobilities of posterior pituitary extracts from human (H-pp), porcine (P-pp), and bovine (B-pp) glands together with those of their purified neurophysins. The upper drawings are from polyacrylamide gel electrophoresis and the lower ones from starch gel electrophoresis. O, origin; F, ion front. (Drawn from the data of Cheng and Friesen, 1972.)

TABLE III—Amino Acid Composition of Human Neurophysins

Amino acid	Major components, NpI				Minor components, NpII	Unresolved mixture
Lys	3[a]	3[b]	3[c]	3[d]	2[a]	3[e]
His	1	1	1	1	1	1
Arg	5	4	4	4	6	5
Asp	8	7	7	7	5	8
Thr	2	2	2	1	2	2
Ser	5	4	4	5	6	5
Glu	11	10	10	9	13	13
Pro	9	7	9	9	5	8
Gly	15	12	12	13	15	14
Ala	12	9	9	12	8	10
½ Cys	14	13	14	14	14	13
Val	4	3	3	2	3	3
Met	0	0	0	0	1	1
Ile	1	1	1	1	1	2
Leu	8	7	7	7	6	8
Tyr	1	1	1	1	1	1
Phe	3	3	3	3	4	3

[a] Cheng and Friesen (1972).
[b] Foss *et al.* (1973).
[c] Capra *et al.* (1974).
[d] Schlesinger *et al.* (1977a).
[e] Legros *et al.* (1970).

tryptophan suggested that the preparation may not have been completely pure (Table III). The NH_2-terminal amino acid was shown to be alanine, and sequence determination of the first 16 NH_2-terminal amino acids showed a marked similarity to bNpI. The COOH-terminal amino acid was leucine, the same as that found in pNpI and bNpI. This neurophysin may represent the hNpI of Capra *et al.* (1974), as the NH_2-terminal sequences of these two are identical, and perhaps also the hNpI of Cheng and Friesen; although, as noted before, there are differences in the amino acid composition of these two. In a later publication (Trygstad *et al.,* 1975), the neurophysin is identified as and designated hNpII, there being a more acidic hormone-binding protein that can be detected in human tissue. In this context, it is noticeable that, in Cheng and Friesen's (1972) paper, a more acidic band can be detected in the starch gel electrophoretic run of pituitary extract, and Robinson (see below), during PAGE of proteins purified from human pituitaries, has a fast running band which, although it is not designated as a major neurophysin shows neurophysinlike immunoreactivity.

Robinson (1975a) prepared a crude neurophysin preparation from acetone-dried, human, posterior pituitaries by classical methods and then further fractionated this material by ion exchange chromatography and by preparative PAGE. The latter method resulted in the separation of four peptides (PGI–IV), all of which were able to bind [4-^{14}C]glycine oxytocin, although the fastest running material did not seem to be a major component in the crude neurophysin preparations (see Fig. 4). The hNpI of Cheng and Friesen runs with a mobility on PAGE similar to the third band of Robinson. An antibody raised to Cheng and Friesen's hNpI cross-reacted with Robinson's PGIII, but not with I, II, and IV, and another antibody showed no cross-reaction with PGIII or the Cheng and Friesen hNpI but recognized PGI, and II and IV. Physiological experiments carried out by Robinson suggest that PGII is a nicotine-stimulated neurophysin and PGIII an estrogen-stimulated neurophysin; these possibly equate to a vasopressin– and to an oxytocin–neurophysin, respectively (see Section V,E).

Watkins (1971) chromatographed an extract of acetone-dried, human glands on Sephadex G-75 and found that his neurophysin-rich eluate showed one major and three minor bands after starch gel electrophoresis.

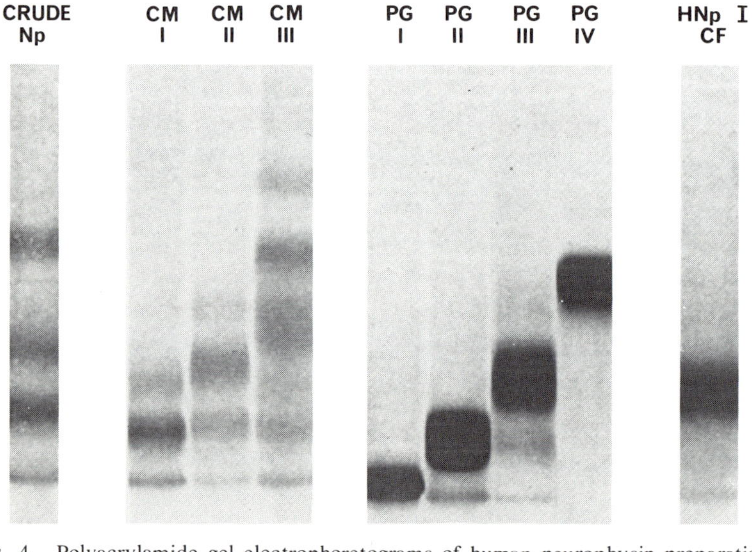

FIG. 4. Polyacrylamide gel electrophoretograms of human neurophysin preparations. Crude Np, neurophysin mixture from Sephadex G-75; CM I-III, proteins resolved by ion-exchange chromatography on CM-Sephadex; PGI-IV, proteins resolved by preparative polyacrylamide gel electrophoresis; HNpI CF; Cheng and Friesen's preparation of hNpI. (From Robinson, 1975a.)

It is evident that the picture in the human is still somewhat unclear, but it appears that there are probably two major neurophysins. On the one hand, Capra's hNpI, Friesen's I-CF, Robinson's PGIII, and Trygstad's II are probably the same, while the second protein is represented by Friesen's II-CF, Robinson's PGIV, and Trygstad's III. This scheme fits with the sparse physiological and sequence data that is at present available. Whether or not the additional bands, e.g., PGI and II of Robinson, are artifacts of extraction or represent the equivalent of the porcine and bovine minor components remains to be elucidated. One lesson which was clearly shown by Hollenberg and Hope (1968) is the importance of avoiding the possibility of proteolytic action during extraction of neurophysins, since the multiplicity of bovine components found by some workers (Hollenberg and Hope, 1967; LaBella *et al.,* 1971) almost certainly resulted from such action. Clearly, it is very difficult to obtain human glands sufficiently soon after death to avoid the possibility of some degradation prior to extraction.

D. RAT

The neurophysins of other species have not been so intensively investigated. The rat has probably received most attention, although the results obtained by different investigators do not yield an unequivocal picture. Pickering and co-workers using analytical and preparative PAGE have been able to separate and purify three rat neurophysins: two major and one minor component. These have been designated A, B, and C on the basis of their mobility, with A being the most anodal (Burford *et al.,* 1971a). All of the three proteins bind the hormones and show an amino acid composition typical of neurophysins. Histidine is probably absent from all three and they all contain one residue/mole of methionine. Watkins (1972a) and Coy and Wuu (1972) have also described the purifications of three rat neurophysins, Watkins using ion-exchange chromatography and Coy and Wuu preparative PAGE. However, both these investigations have shown only one major component and two minor components. The major preparation of both Coy and Wuu (1972) and of Watkins (1972a) contained one residue of methionine and no histidine. Pickering *et al.* (1975) have suggested that, in fact, the single neurophysin component of Watkins (1972a) and of Coy and Wuu (1972) represents an unresolved mixture of the two major peptides that could be separated in the electrophoretic system of Burford and Pickering (1972). Amino acid analysis does allow this explanation, and, in addition, it appears that the peptide III isolated by Coy and Wuu (1972) is very similar in composition to the component designated C by Pickering and colleagues (see Table IV). This

TABLE IV—Amino Acid Composition of Rat Neurophysins

Amino acid	Major components						Minor components			
	Resolved				Unresolved					
	NpA[a]	NpI[b]	NpB[a]	NpII[b]	Protein 11[c]	Np 11[d]	Protein 1[c]	NpC[a]	NpIII[b]	Protein 111[c]
Lys	3	2	3	3	3	3	2	2	3	2
His	0	0	0	0	0	0	0	0	0	0
Arg	6	6	5	5	6	6	5	4	5	4
Asp	5	5	7	8	6	7	5	7	8	6
Thr	3	3	3	3	3	4	2	3	3	3
Ser	7	7	7	7	7	7	7	5	6	5
Glu	13	13	10	10	13	11	14	7	8	8
Pro	8	8	8	10	9	7	8	7	9	8
Gly	13	14	14	15	14	13	14	12	13	13
Ala	9	9	9	9	8	9	8	7	9	8
½ Cys	12	14	12	14	14	12	14	10	13	10
Val	1	1	1	1	1	2	1	1	1	1
Met	1	1	1	1	1	1	1	1	1	1
Ile	2	2	2	2	2	2	2	1	1	2
Leu	6	7	6	7	7	8	7	5	6	5
Tyr	1	1	1	1	1	1	1	1	1	1
Phe	4	4	3	3	3	3	3	2	3	2

[a] Pickering *et al.* (1975) with correction of misprint for Val.
[b] North and Valtin (1977).
[c] Coy and Wuu (1972).
[d] Watkins (1972a).

explanation seems all the more possible now that it is evident that other workers (Sunde and Sokol, 1975; Norström, 1975) have been able to confirm the occurrence of two major and one minor neurophysins if the Burford and Pickering (1972) system is used. This system relies on the high affinity of rat NpA for bromophenol blue, so that during electrophoresis it forms a complex with the dye and, thus, increases its mobility. Very recently, North and Valtin (1977) have also obtained samples of all three rat neurophysins, and their amino acid analyses are in good agreement with those of Pickering and colleagues (Table IV).

E. Ovine

Watkins (1972b; 1973) has isolated one major and two minor neurophysins by ion-exchange chromatography of extracts from acetone-dried sheep posterior pituitary powders. The major component designated oNpIII contained one residue of methionine, but no histidine, while the minor components contained histidine, but lacked methionine. Using fresh-frozen ovine pituitaries, Chrétien and Gilardeau (1973) described a neurophysin prepared by ion-exchange chromatography. The amino acid composition of this was very similar to the component III of Watkins, containing methionine but no histidine (Table V). Alanine was detected at the NH_2-terminus and valine at the COOH-terminus, although PAGE showed that the preparation was not completely homogeneous. Chauvet *et al*. (1975a) have also isolated an ovine neurophysin component which, like the oNp III of Watkins (1973), comprised some 70% of the total neurophysins in the sheep. This major ovine neurophysin contains one residue/mole of methionine and has a sequence very similar to that of bNp II (see Section IV). The presence of a single major neurophysin component in the sheep is interesting and must be borne in mind when considering the possible relationships of the various neurophysin components present in a species.

TABLE V—Amino Acid Composition of Ovine Neurophysins

Amino acid	Minor components		Major component		
	NpI	NpII	NpIII		
Lys	2[a]	2[a]	2[a]	2[b]	2[c]
His	1	1	0	0	0
Arg	6	5	6	7	7
Asp	9	8	5	5	4
Thr	3	3	3	2	2
Ser	8	7	6	6	6
Glu	11	10	14	14	13
Pro	10	8	9	8	8
Gly	16	14	14	14	15
Ala	11	9	7	7	6
½ Cys	14	12	14	12	14
Val	4	3	3	3	3
Met	0	0	1	1	1
Ile	2	2	4	3	4
Leu	8	7	7	6	6
Tyr	1	1	1	1	1
Phe	4	3	3	3	3

[a] Watkins (1973).
[b] Chrétien and Gilardeau (1973).
[c] From sequence of Chauvet *et al*. (1975b).

F. Guinea Pig

Like the sheep it appears that, at least for the present, only one major neurophysin can be detected. Watkins and Ellis (1973) suggest that the guinea pig has only one major and possibly one minor neurophysin component. Amino acid analysis of the major component showed a protein with the characteristics of a neurophysin but containing neither methionine nor histidine. Sachs *et al.* (1971a, 1975) have also isolated only one major neurophysin component from the guinea pig, and this single component could not be further resolved by PAGE in the presence of bromphenol blue or by isoelectric focusing. The amino acid composition of the guinea pig neurophysin isolated by Sachs and his group shows slight differences from that obtained by Watkins although these are not great (see Table VI). The main noticeable difference is the presence of histidine in Sachs' guinea pig neurophysin.

TABLE VI—Amino Acid Composition of a Guinea Pig Neurophysin

Amino acid	Major components	
Lys	1[a]	1[b]
His	0	1
Arg	4	5
Asp	7	5
Thr	3	2
Ser	4	4
Glu	12	11
Pro	7	6
Gly	10	10
Ala	7	6
½ Cys	12	14
Val	3	3
Met	0	0
Ile	1	1
Leu	6	5
Tyr	1	1
Phe	3	2

[a] Watkins and Ellis (1973).
[b] Sachs *et al.* (1975).

G. Fish

Pickering (1968) isolated a hormone-binding protein from acetone-dried cod pituitaries by gel filtration and DEAE–Sephadex chromatography. The amino acid composition of this protein is remarkably similar to that of the mammalian neurophysins (see Table VII), and the maintenance of such close similarity, at least throughout the vertebrate phylum, argues for a physiological role for the neurophysins.

TABLE VII—Amino Acid Composition of Cod Neurophysin[a]

Amino acid	Component
Lys	2
His	1
Arg	4
Asp	7
Thr	3
Ser	8
Glu	16
Pro	9
Gly	15
Ala	9
$\frac{1}{2}$ Cys	11
Val	3
Met	1
Ile	2
Leu	9
Tyr	1
Phe	2

[a] Calculated from Pickering (1968) assuming an MW of 10,000.

IV. Structure of Neurophysins

The striking similarity in the amino acid composition of the neurophysins of many species is evident from the preceding section. In the last few years, the advent of modern automatic sequencing techniques coupled with advances in separation methods has enabled the structure of a number of neurophysins to be elucidated. To date, there are available complete or partial sequences for two bovine (Walter *et al.*, 1971; Capra *et al.*, 1972; Schlesinger *et al.*, 1972; North *et al.*, 1975; Wuu and Crumm, 1976a; Chauvet *et al.*, 1976), three porcine (Wuu *et al.*, 1971; Wuu and Crumm, 1973, 1976b), one human (Foss *et al.*, 1973; Capra *et al.*, 1974; Schlesinger *et al.*, 1977a), one ovine (Chauvet *et al.*, 1975a,b, 1976) 2 dog (Walter *et al.*, 1977), 2 rat (Walter and Audhya, 1977), 2 guinea pig (Schlesinger *et al.*, 1977b), and one cod (Schlesinger *et al.*, 1977b) neurophysins, and Fig. 5 compares the available sequence data.

Overall, there is a large degree of homology between the various neurophysins although definite differences can be discerned. In general terms, the central part of each molecule shows least variation, while the first nine amino acids and those in the COOH-terminal quarter of the molecule are subject to most variations.

Looking first at the bovine neurophysins the main features noted are as follows: bNpI differs from bNpII in 5 of the first 9 amino acids and in 14 of the last 25 residues. There is, however, a large region from residues 10 to 74 in which the two molecules show complete identity.

A suggested assignment of the S–S bonds in bNpI taken from North *et al.* (1975) is shown in Fig. 2. The first suggestions for disulfide assignment in a neurophysin molecule were made for bNpII (Schlesinger *et al.*, 1972), but these are being reassessed in the light of corrected sequences for this molecule suggested by Wuu and Crumm (1976a) and Chauvet *et al.* (1976).

The sequence of porcine NpI is identical to that of bNpII, except for three substitutions at the carboxy terminus. Indeed, the COOH-terminal sequence of pNpI is identical to that of bNpI: Ala-Ser-Phe-Leu-OH. The sequence of hNpI (North *et al.*, 1975; Schlesinger *et al.*, 1977a) shows remarkable similarity to that of bNpI with substitutions at only seven positions (2, 3, 9, 25, 29, 30, 81) in the sequence of 92 residues.

[Very recently, partial sequences for guinea pig and cod neurophysins have been reported (Schlesinger *et al.*, 1977b) and, again, the variations are largely confined to the first nine residues. Interestingly, the sequence of the first 15 residues of cod neurophysin differs from that of bNp II in only three positions: a substitution of Leu for Met at position 2; of Ala for Ser at position 3; and of Gly for Leu at position 5.]

Recently, two groups have provided the complete amino acid sequence for the major ovine neurophysin component (Schlesinger *et al.*, 1975; Chauvet *et al.*, 1975b, 1976). The sequence shown in Fig. 5 is that given by Chauvet *et al.* (1975b, 1976) but is almost identical with that of Schlesinger *et al.* (1975), except for the presence of an extra arginine. The American workers using Watkins's (1972b) preparation found the molecule to consist of 94 residues and to terminate -Pro-Arg-Val-OH, whereas the French group deduced that their protein was 95 residues long and terminated -Pro-Arg-Arg-Val-OH. Moreover, Schlesinger *et al.* found 75–79 to be Asn-Ser-Glu-Ala-Cys, instead of Asn-Asp-Glu-Ser-Cys reported by Chauvet *et al.* As can be seen from Fig. 5, the sequence of the ovine protein is almost identical with that of bNpII and differs only by an Ile/Asn substitution at position 48. The microheterogenicity found at position 89

	1									10										20					
Bovine Np II	Ala	Met	Ser	Asp	Leu	Glu	Leu	Arg	Gln	Cys	Leu	Pro	Cys	Gly	Pro	Gly	Gly	Lys	Gly	Arg	Cys	Phe	Gly	Pro	Ser
Porcine Np I	—	—	—	—	—	—	—	—	—	—	—	—	—	—	—	—	—	—	—	—	—	—	—	—	—
Ovine Np	—	—	—	—	—	—	—	—	—	—	—	—	—	—	—	—	—	—	—	—	—	—	—	—	—
Bovine Np I	—	Val	Leu	—	—	Asp	Val	—	Thr	—	—	—	—	—	—	—	—	—	—	—	—	—	—	—	—
Human Np I	—	Ala	Pro	—	—	Asp	Val	—	Lys	—	—	—	—	—	—	—	—	—	—	—	—	—	—	—	Asn
Rat Np I (A)	—	Ala	Leu	—	—	Asp	Met	—	Lys	—	—	—	—	—	—	—	—	—	—	—	—	—	—	—	—
Rat Np II (B)	—	Thr	—	—	Met	—	—	—	—	—	—	—	—	—	—	—	—	—	—	—	—	—	—	—	—
Dog Np I	—	Ala	Leu	—	—	Asp	Val	—	—	—	—	—	—	—	—	—	—	Gln	—						
Dog Np II	—	—	—	—	—	—	—																		

					30										40										50
Bovine Np II	Ile	Cys	Cys	Gly	Asp	Glu	Leu	Gly	Cys	Phe	Val	Gly	Thr	Ala	Glu	Ala	Leu	Arg	Cys	Gln	Glu	Glu	Asn	Tyr	Leu
Porcine Np I	—	—	—	—	—	—	—	—	—	—	—	—	—	—	—	—	—	—	—	—	—	—	—	—	—
Ovine Np	—	—	—	—	—	—	—	—	—	—	—	—	—	—	—	—	—	—	—	—	—	—	Ile	—	—
Bovine Np I	—	—	—	—	—	—	—	—	—	—	—	—	—	—	—	—	—	—	—	—	—	—	—	—	—
Human Np I	—	—	—	Ala	Glu	—	—	—	—	—	—	—	—	—	—	—	—	—	—	—	—	—	—	—	—
Rat Np I (A)	—	—	—	Ala	—	—	—	—	—	—	—	—	—	—	—	—	—	—	—	—	—	—	—	—	—
Rat Np II (B)	—	—	—	Ala	—	—	—	—	—	—	—	—	—	—	—	—	—	—	—	—	—	—	—	—	—

										60										70					
Bovine Np II	Pro	Ser	Pro	Cys	Gln	Ser	Gly	Gln	Lys	Pro	Cys	Gly	Ser	Gly	Gly	Arg	Cys	Ala	Ala	Ala	Gly	Ile	Cys	Cys	Asn
Porcine Np I	—	—	—	—	—	—	—	—	—	—	—	—	—	—	—	—	—	—	—	—	—	—	—	—	—
Ovine Np	—	—	—	—	—	—	—	—	—	—	—	—	—	—	—	—	—	—	—	—	—	—	—	—	—
Bovine Np I	—	—	—	—	—	—	—	—	—	—	—	—	—	—	—	—	—	—	—	—	—	—	—	—	Ser
Human Np I	—	—	—	—	—	—	—	—	—	Ala	—	—	—	—	—	—	—	—	—	—	—	Leu	—	—	Ser

					80									Val	90					95
Bovine Np II	Asp	Glu	Ser	Cys	Val	Thr	Glu	Pro	Glu	Cys	Arg	Glu	Gly	Ile	Gly	Phe	Pro	Arg	Arg	Val
Porcine Np I	—	—	—	—	—	—	—	—	—	—	—	—	—	Ala	Ser	—	Leu (92)			
Ovine Np	—	—	—	—	—	—	—	—	—	—	—	—	—	Ile	—	—	—	—	—	— (95)
Bovine Np I	Pro	Asp	Gly	—	His	Glu	Asp	—	Ala	—	Asp	Pro	Glu	Ala	Ser	—	Leu (92)			
Human Np I	Pro	Asp	Gly	—	His	Ala	Asp	—	Ala	—	Asp	Pro	Glu	Ala	Ser	—	Leu (92)			

FIG. 5. Comparison of the available sequences for neurophysins. Data for bNpII from Wuu and Crumm (1976a), Chauvet *et al.* (1976); pNpI, Wuu *et al.* (1971); oNp, Chauvet *et al.* (1975b); bNpI and hNpI, Schlesinger *et al.* (1977a); rNpI and II, Walter and Audhya (1977); dog Np, Walter *et al.* (1977).

in the bovine peptide (Wuu and Crumm, 1976a; Chauvet *et al.*, 1976), which is either Val or Ile, is not apparent in the ovine peptide.

On structural terms, two groups of neurophysin peptides seem to be discernible. Those with NH_2-terminal sequences similar to bNpI and those with sequences similar to bNpII. Chauvet *et al.* (1975a,b) argue for the abolition of a nomenclature based on electrophoretic mobility and its replacement by one based on the amino acids present as residues 2, 3, 6, 7. Thus, one group would consist of the proteins bNpII, pNpI, and oNpIII which have Met, Ser, Glu, Leu at positions 2, 3, 6, and 7, respectively (called MSEL–neurophysins by Chauvet *et al.*), and the other group (called VLDV–neurophysins by Chauvet *et al.*), at present comprising bNpI and pNpII, which has Val, Leu, Asp, Val in these positions. [Chauvet *et al.* (1975a) quote a partial sequence for pNpII attributed to Wuu and Crumm (1973), but this is not recorded in their abstract.] Considering the bovine and porcine neurophysins alone, it is tempting to suggest a functional significance for the two groups of neurophysins, since in these species it would appear that the MSEL–neurophysins are associated with vasopressin and the VLDV–neurophysins with oxytocin (see Section V,C). However, hNpI which, although not a typical VLDV protein, does not fall into the MSEL group seems to be associated with vasopressin. Moreover, all three rat neurophysins appear to contain methionine, and their NH_2-terminal sequences (Walter and Audhya, 1977) do not allow them to be classified by the nomenclature of Acher and his colleagues. The recently determined partial sequences of guinea pig and cod neurophysins (Schlesinger *et al.*, 1977b) are also outside of the Acher nomenclature. Thus, we must await further elucidation both of structure and of hormone association for the neurophysins of other species before we can determine whether the neurophysins can be classified in structural groups having functional significance.

Study of the invariance of several residues in the different neurophysin proteins (Fig. 6) provides information on the possible correlations between structure and function. The positions of glycine and proline residues are noticeably preserved: 12 glycine residues are found in identical positions in those proteins which have been sequenced. Similarly, eight proline residues hold invariate positions. A strongly hydrophobic region exists from residues 10 to 38, and this contains many of the invariant glycines and prolines. The region from residues 38 to 57 appears to be almost invariant in all of the neurophysins studied (Gly/Ala at 29, Glu/Asp at 30, and in oNpIII Ile/Asn substitution at 48), but it contains few hydrophobic residues. Furthermore, it contains the region (42–44) that is most susceptible to tryptic and chymotryptic cleavage (Capra and Walter, 1975) and, as Capra and Walter suggest, may indicate that this region represents

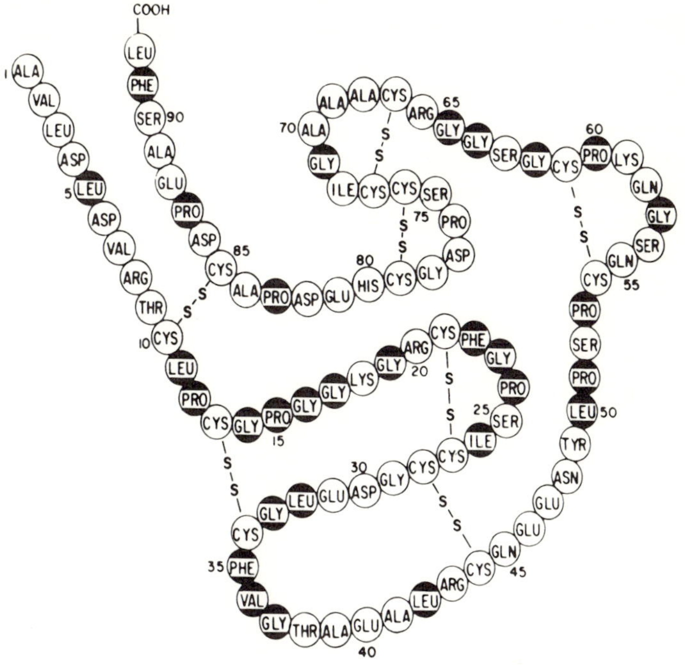

FIG. 6. The positions of the glycine, proline, and hydrophobic amino acids which are invariant among the neurophysin sequences presently available. (From Capra and Walter, 1975, and Schlesinger *et al.*, 1977a.)

the polar surface of the molecule, which is involved in the nonapeptide-binding phenomena. This idea is consistent with evidence suggesting that the Tyr^{49} is in close proximity to Tyr^{2} of the peptide in protein–ligand interactions (see Section VI,A).

A. Molecular Weight Heterogeneity

Estimates of the MW of bovine and porcine neurophysins have shown considerable variations. Ultracentrifugation studies indicated that the MW of the bovine protein–hormone complex isolated by van Dyke *et al.* (1942) was about 30,000. Similarly Ginsburg and Ireland (1965) estimated that their preparation of bovine neurophysin prepared from fresh material had an MW of 25,000. Equilibrium sedimentation studies led Hollenberg and Hope (1968) to believe that the MW of the bovine neurophysins I and II that they had isolated were of the order of 20,000. The porcine neurophysin preparation prepared by Ginsburg *et al.* (1966) appeared to be similar to their bovine neurophysin preparations with an MW of

25,000. Later investigations of the same material by the same group (Ginsburg and Thomas, 1969) using gel filtration and sedimentation equilibrium methods gave a value of 13,000 for the MW. Friesen and Astwood (1967) obtained a value of 25,000 for their porcine NpI preparations, whereas the equivalent material isolated by Wuu and Saffran (1969b) and by Rudman *et al.* (1970) had MW of less than 10,000.

Consideration of binding isotherm data led Ginsburg and Thomas (1969) to suggest that porcine neurophysin might be a polymerizing equilibrium system, and this view has since been confirmed. Uttenthal and Hope (1970) estimated the weight average MW of pNpI and pNpII at low pH and found that these were concentration-dependent, obtaining values of 1.7–2.2 times the monomer MW, with protein concentrations varying from 1.4 to 4.0 mg/ml. Burford *et al.* (1969) showed, by zonal and frontal analysis of the elution pattern obtained during the gel filtration of porcine neurophysin, that the protein was an aggregating system which rapidly reached equilibrium. These authors later confirmed their findings (Burford *et al.,* 1971b) and showed that the weight-average MW of their porcine neurophysin prepared from fresh glands was concentration-dependent. An increase in protein concentration from 1 to 7 mg/ml at pH 5.8 increased the weight-average MW from approximately 10,000 to 35,000. Moreover, Burford *et al*. (1971b) found that the equilibrium was perturbed by calcium ions. At pH 5.8, addition of calcium to 10^{-5} *M* stabilized the weight-average MW of their preparation at 21,000 irrespective of protein concentration. This is an interesting finding since this group of workers also find an effect of Ca^{2+} in the binding of hormones to neurophysin—a phenomenon which has not been confirmed by other workers using different preparations of porcine neurophysin (see Section VI,B).

In bovine neurophysins, too, the studies of Breslow *et al.* (1971) showed that the sedimentation coefficient of bNpII was dependent on protein concentration in a manner suggestive of a self-associating system. Their sedimentation-equilibrium studies indicated that both bNpI and bNpII showed MW heterogeneities and that simple monomer–dimer equilibrium adequately described the results.

There is, therefore, strong evidence that the bovine and porcine neurophysins, and presumably those of other species too, can form a self-aggregating system, dependent on such factors as protein concentration, pH, ionic strength, and presence of neurohypophyseal peptide or Ca^{2+} ions. The physiological significance of this is not clear, but one possibility suggested by Burford *et al.* (1971b) is that, at intragranular concentrations, the relatively low abundance of the monomeric form, whether or not complexed with hormone, would tend to be low and so would reduce the potential osmotic effect of the intragranular protein.

This suggestion can only be tentative, however, until much more is known about the intragranular form and environment of the neurophysins, especially since the available evidence tends to suggest that the granular constituents are present in the solid phase rather than in solution (Morris and Cannata, 1973; Morris, 1976).

B. The Native Form

Studies of the histochemical properties and composition of a variety of storage and secretory organelles has led to the suggestion that soluble, acidic lipoproteins constitute a significant component of their internal matrices (Koenig, 1974). There is also a body of experimental evidence which suggests that the neurophysins in their natural state, at least, may be members of this group of proteins which all seem to be intimately associated in the storage granule with the eventual secretory products.

Potassium bromide ultracentrifugal flotation of a bovine NSG lysate preparation resulted in the separation of high density lipoprotein (HDLP) and very high density lipoprotein (VHDLP) fractions, the former being enriched in phospholipid, protein, and cholesterol (Mylroie and Koenig, 1971). The inability of dialysis to dissociate the lipid and protein constituents of these preparations indicated that there was some form of complex formation between the lipid and protein moieties. Amino acid analysis of both of these lipoprotein fractions revealed an amino acid composition, which resembled that of the neurophysins (Mylroie and Koenig, 1971), being rich in glutamic acid, glycine, proline, and cysteine (see Table VIII). Polyacrylamide gel electrophoresis of the HDLP and VHDLP fractions, as well as of a total Triton X-100 extract of the NSG showed two major protein bands that had R_f's very similar to those of the major bovine neurophysins. In addition, the two major bands derived from the lipoprotein fractions stained weakly with the lipophylic stain Sudan Black-B as well, as revealing their acidic nature by staining metachromatically with acridine orange. Chloroform–methanol extraction of the gels prior to staining abolished the reaction with the lipid stains, although the metachromatic acridine orange staining was retained. Labeling experiments in the rat *in vivo* involving the intraventricular administration of ^{3}H-labeled myoinositol (Koenig and Mylroie, 1975) showed that the label was associated with the rat neurophysin region when the radioactive neural lobe extracts were subjected to PAGE and to isoelectric focusing.

Confirmation for these ideas has come from work carried out by Pliška and co-workers. Their interest in the subject was initially stimulated by their hormone-binding experiments utilizing agarose-bound neurophysin

TABLE VIII—Comparison of the Composition of the Bovine Neurophysins with that of the Lipoproteins from Bovine NSG

Amino acid	Bovine[a] neurophysins		Lipoprotein[b] fractions	
	NpI	NpII	HDLP	VHDLP
Lys	2	2	4	3
His	1	0	1	1
Arg	4	7	7	7
Asp	7	5	8	8
Thr	2	2	4	3
Ser	5	6	6	7
Glu	11	14	14	13
Pro	9	8	7	8
Gly	14	16	13	14
Ala	9	6	9	8
$\frac{1}{2}$ Cys	14	14	6	11
Val	3	4	5	4
Met	0	1	1	1
Ile	2	2	3	3
Leu	6	6	8	7
Tyr	1	1	2	2
Phe	3	3	4	3

[a] Breslow *et al.* (1971).
[b] Calculated from Koenig and Mylroie (1975).

(Pliška and Sachs, 1974). Using this preparation, they were able to demonstrate the presence of more than one population of binding sites with differing affinities, while most other investigators were able to detect only low-affinity binding sites (see Section IV,B). Earlier studies (Ginsburg and Ireland, 1965; Ginsburg and Thomas, 1969), in which relatively crude neurophysin prepared from fresh bovine glands was used, indicated the presence of only high-affinity hormone binding sites, so that it seemed that these differences shown by the various neurophysin preparations might be a function of the method of their preparation.

Pliška and Meyer-Grass (1975) prepared bovine NSG and disrupted them by sonication in Triton X-100 to obtain a crude lysate. Chromatography of the lysate on Sephadex G-25 gave a protein fraction which showed the presence of only two main components on PAGE, and these had R_f's identical to those of bovine neurophysins I and II. Preparative PAGE enabled the purification of this bNpI and II of granular origin.

Amino acid analysis of these two proteins showed that they had an amino acid composition very similar to (but not completely identical with) bNpI and bNpII prepared by other investigators using more conventional extraction methods. Analysis of the proteins also revealed the presence of 10–20 hexosamine residues per mole, and these were mainly present in the form of glucosamine. It is interesting to note that Hvas and Thorn (1973) were also able to detect hexosamine in their preparation of bovine NSG's. As a further step, the proteins of the NSG lysate separated by PAGE were eluted from the gel and extracted in organic lipid solvents. The dried extracts were examined by gas–liquid chromatography mass spectrometry after derivatization, and all the extracts from the granular bNpI and bNpII were found to contain two saturated fatty acids—stearic and palmitic. Pliška and Meyer-Grass (1975) comment that the lipid binding to the protein (or carbohydrate present) must be very weak, as mild acidic conditions are sufficient to disrupt it.

Immunologically, the NSG-derived neurophysins reacted essentially like the conventionally prepared neurophysins. Hormone-binding experiments, however, indicated that the granular neurophysins had only one population of binding sites, and this was of the high-affinity type. Also, and perhaps more significantly, strong acid or alkali treatment converted the binding properties of the NSG lysate neurophysins to values similar to those found for the conventionally prepared neurophysin.

Thus, there is increasing evidence that the neurophysins may themselves be, or may be closely associated with, lipoproteins or glycolipoproteins. Jones and Swann (1974, 1975) have presented radiolabeling evidence for a fucose-containing material, possibly a peptide of about 10,000 MW present in rat NSG, but this appears to be distinguishable from the rat neurophysins. The function of such a peptide, which may be analogous to the glycopeptides isolated from porcine posterior pituitary powders by Holwerda (1972), and its relation to the neurophysins, remains to be elucidated. Evidence is also accumulating to suggest that the real native structure of the neurophysin present in the neurosecretory granules *in vivo* may not be the same as that of the neurophysins, which have been subjected to intensive purification procedures. Even the low pH technique initiated by Dean and Hope (1968) to minimize proteolysis during extraction may modify the native form by stripping loosely bound lipid and sugar moieties from the molecule. Perhaps, at this juncture in the study of neurophysins, it may be well to heed the conclusion of Pliška and Meyer-Grass (1975) . . . "any discussion of the biological role of the neurophysins based on the properties of the conventional preparations may be at least speculative, and at worst misleading."

V. Relationship of Hormones and Neurophysins

A. Neurophysins as Carrier Proteins

The concept of neurosecretion originally proposed by E. Scharrer (see Scharrer and Scharrer, 1954) and applied to the vertebrate hypothalamo-neurohypohyseal system by Bargmann (1949) holds that the hormones oxytocin and vasopressin are synthesized in neurons whose perikarya reside in the paraventricular and supraoptic nuclei of the hypothalamus, and are then transported along the axons of these neurons for storage in, and release from, their nerve endings in the neural lobe of the pituitary gland. The evidence that the posterior pituitary hormones were neurosecretory products was largely histological and came from the application of specific stains (later shown to be staining mainly the neurophysins (Acher, 1958) to the study of sections of the hypothalamus and neurophpophysis after animals had been subjected to stimuli known to bring about the release of oxytocin and/or vasopressin (Hild, 1951; Hild and Zetler, 1953a,b; Sloper, 1954, 1955). In 1957, Palay described the ultrastructure of the neurohypophysis and drew attention to the abundance of electron-dense granules within dilatations of the axon terminals of the hypothalamo-neurohypophyseal tract. These granules, thereafter called neurosecretory granules (NSG), were very soon obtained in a purified form by differential centrifugation of homogenates of the neural lobe, and shown to be the store for a very large proportion of the oxytocin and vasopressin present in the gland (Lederis and Heller, 1960; Weinstein *et al.,* 1961; Barer *et al.,* 1963; LaBella *et al.,* 1963; Dean and Hope, 1967). The neurophysins had been characterized as neurohypophyseal proteins which bound the hormones with high specificity, and once it became established that the hormones were products of neurosecretion, it seemed natural to regard the neurophysins as carrier proteins with the function of binding the hormones during their intraneuronal transport (Sawyer, 1961; Ginsburg, 1968; Jongkind, 1972). Certainly, they are present within NSG (Ginsburg and Ireland, 1966; Dean and Hope, 1967), and so could well perform this function, although it now appears that their relationship with the hormones may be more intimate than this.

B. Parallel Release of Hormones and Neurophysins

The development of radioimmunoassays for the neurophysins (Martin *et al.,* 1972; Cheng and Friesen, 1973; Legros *et al.,* 1969) allowed the demonstration that the release of neurophypophyseal hormone *in vivo* or *in vitro* was always accompanied by neurophysin release (Uttenthal *et al.,*

1971; Legros *et al.,* 1971; McNeilly *et al.,* 1972). Although it was possible to show, in some cases, that release occurred in constant proportions (e.g., see Nordmann *et al.,* 1971; Matthews *et al.,* 1973) the use of animals or glands from one species and purified neurophysin, as both standard and antigen, from another precluded the determination of the precise quantitative relationship between the amounts of hormone and neurophysin released.

C. Association of Oxytocin and Vasopressin with Separate Neurophysins

When Hope and his colleagues (Hollenberg and Hope, 1968; Dean and Hope, 1968) showed that the large number of bovine neurophysins obtained by earlier workers probably resulted from enzymic activity during extraction, and that the bovine posterior pituitary contained only two native neurophysins in any measure of abundance, it seemed pertinent to ask if each hormone had its own specific neurophysin. Certainly, the neurophysin molecules themselves show no specificity of binding as has been discussed above, but is there a specific association *in vivo?* The first indication that there might be came from the observation (Dean *et al.,* 1968a) that, during isopyknic centrifugation of bovine NSG's, bovine NpI tended to sediment along with oxytocin and NpII with vasopressin. At the same time, Hope and his colleagues (Dean *et al.,* 1968b) reported data which, reinterpreted in the light of our present knowledge of the MW of the protein, showed that the bovine posterior pituitary contained approximately 1 mole of oxytocin per mole of bovine NpI and 1 mole of vasopressin per mole of bovine NpII. With the development of specific radioimmunoassays for the individual bovine neurophysins (Robinson *et al.,* 1971a), it became possible to measure the changes in the blood concentration of the proteins, and it was found that conditions and stimuli associated with the release of oxytocin (e.g., parturition, milking) led to a preferential release of bovine NpI, whereas those which were associated with the release of vasopressin (e.g., dehydration, hemorrhage) led to a preferential release of bovine NpII (Robinson *et al.,* 1971b; Legros *et al.,* 1974, 1975b).

In common with many other species (see above), the rat also contains in its neurohypophysis two major neurophysin proteins that can be separated by polyacrylamide gel electrophoresis (Rennels, 1966; Friesen and Astwood, 1967; Burford and Pickering, 1971). One of these (the one with the higher electrophoretic mobility) is absent (Burford *et al.,* 1971a) from animals that are homozygous for diabetes insipidus and known (Valtin *et al.,* 1965) to be unable to synthesize vasopressin. The rat neurophysins

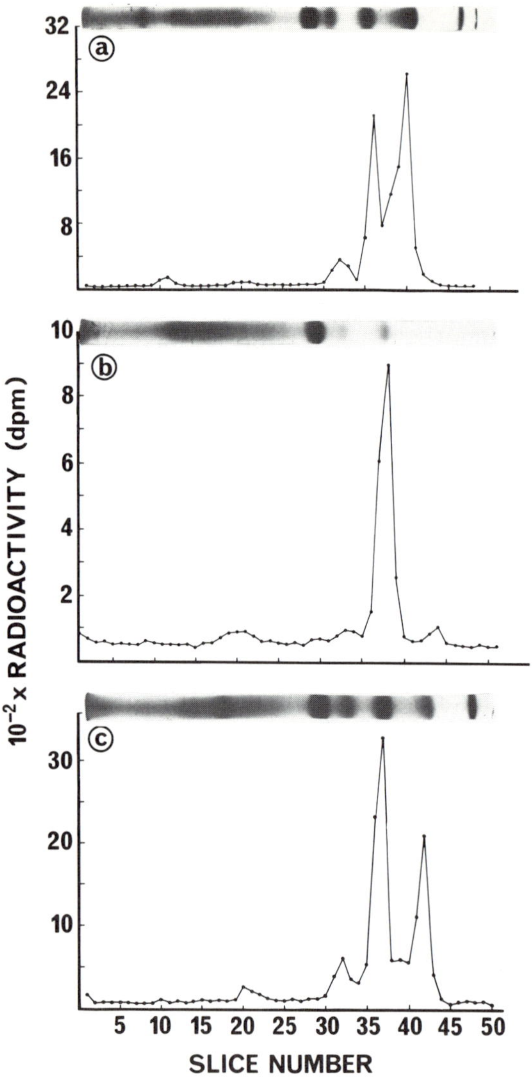

FIG. 7. The distribution of radioactivity 24 hours after intracisternal injection of ^{35}S-labeled cysteine, among the neurophysins on polyacrylamide gel columns after electrophoresis of gland extracts from (a) normal, (b) homozygous, and (c) heterozygous Brattleboro rats. Note absence of the second neurophysin peak in the homozygous rats with severe diabetes insipidus. (From Cross *et al.*, 1975.)

can be radioactively labeled *in vivo* by giving the animals subarachnoid injections of ^{35}S-labeled cysteine. It can then be readily demonstrated (Fig. 7) that the neurophysin, which is absent from homozygous Brattleboro rats, is present in smaller amounts than the other major component in the glands of heterozygous Brattleboros, which contain more oxytocin than vasopressin, and in larger amounts in the glands of normal animals. Moreover, the ratio of radioactivity in NpA to that in NpB is the same as the ratio of vasopressin/oxytocin in the glands of all three types, provided that they are examined within 24 hours of labeling (see below). On the basis of these findings, it was suggested that NpA, which by conventional nomenclature would be rat NpI, is associated with vasopressin and that NpB (rat NpII) is associated with oxytocin (Burford *et al.*, 1971a). Preliminary results have indicated that there is an approximately 1 : 1 relationship between the amounts of NpA and vasopressin stored in normal and Brattleboro rat glands (Pickering *et al.*, 1975).

It came as something of a surprise to find that, in the rat, it was the neurophysin with the higher mobility which appeared to be vasopressin-linked, since it had become accepted, from unwarranted extrapolation by other workers of the findings of Hope and his colleagues, that NpI was the oxytocin-linked protein and NpII the vasopressin-linked one in all species, and it was for this reason that the A, B, C terminology was introduced. Ironically, now that indications of specific hormone association exist in four species (ox, pig, rat, and human) it is the bovine proteins which are out of step at present (Table IX). Isopyknic centrifugation of NSG's from pig glands have shown (Pickup *et al.*, 1973) that porcine NpI tends to sediment along with vasopressin and porcine NpII with oxytocin. In humans, too, it would appear that human NpI is associated with vasopressin and human NpII with oxytocin, since the latter was essentially absent from an oat cell carcinoma that was secreting vasopressin without oxytocin, but present in one which produced both hormones (Legros and Louis,

TABLE IX—Hormone Associated Neurophysins[a] in Different Species

	Neurophysin associated with		
Species	Oxytocin	Vasopressin	Reference
Ox	NpI	NpII	Dean *et al.* (1968a)
Pig	NpII	NpI, NpIII	Pickup *et al.* (1973)
Rat	NpII, NpIII	NpI	Burford *et al.* (1971a)
Human	NpII	NpI	Legros and Louis (1974)

[a] In each case the neurophysins are classified according to electrophoretic mobility.

1974). At present there is only one species, the guinea pig, in which two hormones but only a single major neurophysin have been detected (Sachs *et al.*, 1971a; Watkins and Ellis, 1973). It remains to be shown whether this is because only one protein is synthesized or because the available methods are not adequate for the separation of a vasopressin-neurophysin from an oxytocin-neurophysin in this species.

D. Biosynthesis and Intraneuronal Transport of Hormones and Neurophysins

Sachs and his colleagues have found evidence for the existence of an intermediate inactive protein in the biosynthetic pathway leading to the synthesis of vasopressin (Sachs, 1969, 1970, 1971; Sachs *et al.*, 1969). They showed that during the biosynthesis of vasopressin in both the dog and the guinea pig, *in vivo* and *in vitro*, there is a lag period of some 1–1½ hours before labeled cysteine becomes incorporated into labeled vasopressin and that the events during the lag period are sensitive to protein synthesis inhibitors (e.g., puromycin), while those following the lag period are not (Sachs and Takabatake, 1964; Takabatake and Sachs, 1964). In the same way, Sachs and his colleagues (Sachs *et al.*, 1969, 1971b) showed that neurophysin was also synthesized by way of a precursor and that the "maturation" of this precursor was insensitive to puromycin. As shown in Fig. 8, when pieces of hypothalamic–median eminence tissue taken, from dogs which had received infusions of ^{35}S-labeled cysteine for 1½ hours *in vivo*, were incubated *in vitro* for a further 4.5 hours, there was a considerable increase in the amount of radioactive vasopressin and neurophysin produced during the incubation. Moreover, this accumulation could occur in the absence of protein synthesis (Sachs *et al.*, 1971b).

In the rat (Fig. 9) radioactivity begins to appear in the major neurophysins of the neural lobe between 1 and 2 hours after presentation of ^{35}S-labeled cysteine to the hypothalamus (Norström and Sjöstrand, 1971; Burford and Pickering, 1973) which, taking the length of the tract to be about 3 mm (Sloper, 1958), gives a minimum transport velocity of 1–3 mm/hour. The build up and fall-off of radioactivity in the neural lobe associated with the two major neurophysins exactly parallels that found (Jones and Pickering, 1970, 1972) for oxytocin and vasopressin and, indeed, parallels the changes in radioactivity of the NSG as a whole or their contents and membrane considered separately (Swann and Pickering, 1974a,b, 1976). Thus, it would appear that the hormones and neurophysins are synthesized and transported as an integral unit. There is some disagreement about whether there are one or more rates at which neurophysin is transported along the axons of the hypo-

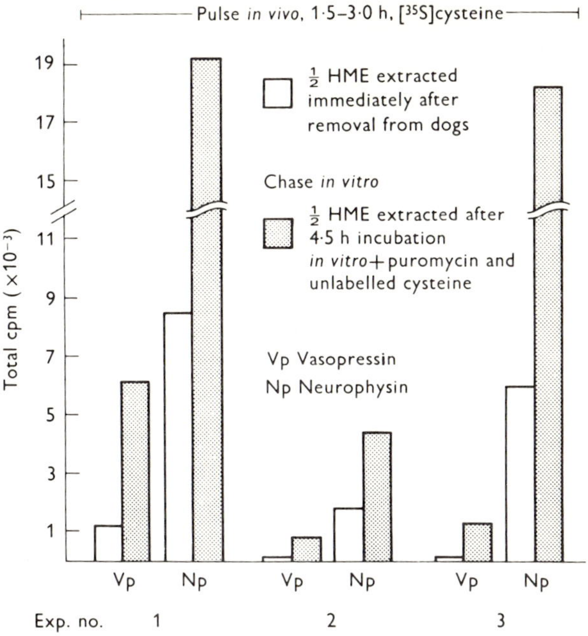

FIG. 8. Production of ^{35}S-labeled vasopressin and neurophysin *in vitro* from dog HME tissues labeled *in vivo*. ^{35}S-labeled cysteine, approximately 1.3–1.7 × 10^9 cpm, was infused into the third ventricle of dogs for 1.5 hours (expts. 1, 2) or 3.0 hours (expt. 3); the dogs were killed, and the HME was excised, divided in the medial plane and one-half was used for the immediate isolation of vasopressin and neurophysin, whereas the other half was sliced and incubated *in vitro* for an additional 4.5 hours. (From Sachs *et al.*, 1971b.)

thalamoneurohypophyseal tract. The Swedish group (Norström and Sjöstrand, 1971; Norström, 1974, 1975) have interpreted their evidence to suggest that there are at least two rates of transport, a rapid one with a velocity akin to that discussed above and a slower one of some 0.5 mm/day, which they equate with the passive transport of neurophysin by the process of axoplasmic flow described by Weiss (1944, 1968). On the other hand, we believe that the "wobbles" in the time-course (e.g., Fig. 9) represent experimental variation, and that the results are consistent with a single rapid phase of transport for the neurophysin within NSG (Burford and Pickering, 1973; Pickering *et al.*, 1974, 1975).

It seems reasonable to suggest that biosynthesis in the rat follows a similar course to that shown by Sachs *et al.* 1969 for the dog and guinea pig and, moreover, that the time required for the synthesis and "maturation" of the precursor in the rat will not be very different from the 1 hour found by Takabatake and Sachs (1964) for the guinea pig. This being so, the results discussed above and shown in Fig. 9, i.e., that radioactive hormones and

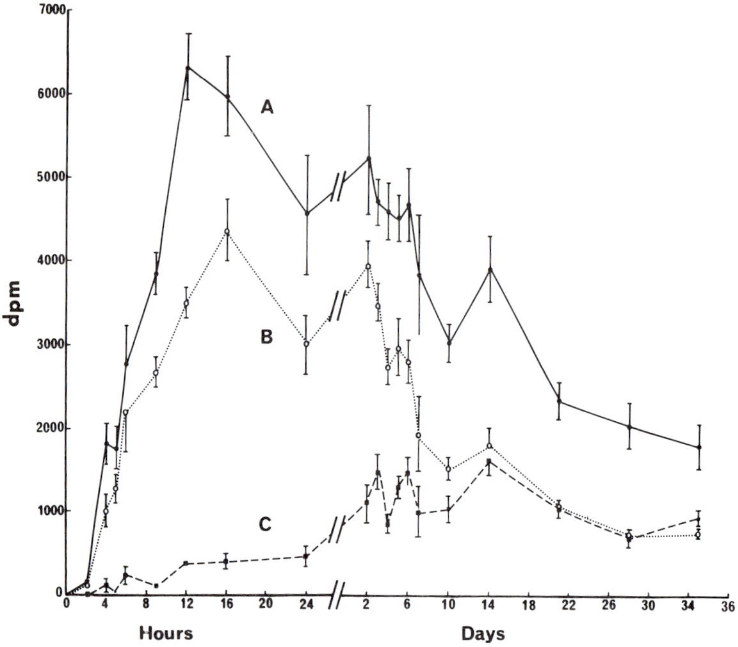

FIG. 9. The change in the radioactivity associated with the three neurophysins (A,B,C) in the neural lobe of the rat resulting from an intracisternal injection of 50 μCi of ^{35}S-labeled cysteine. (From Pickering *et al.*, 1975.)

neurophysins appear in the neural lobe between 1 and 2 hours after injection of radioactive amino acid, suggest *either* that transport is very much faster than 3 mm/hour *or* that the final stages of maturation occur inside the NSG, as they are being transported along the axon. The latter possibility has been suggested before (Vogt, 1953; Sachs *et al.,* 1969; Lederis and Jayasena, 1970; Pickering *et al.,* 1971) and raises the question of the nature of the link between the biosynthesis of the hormones and that of the neurophysin.

With the evidence that both hormones and neurophysins are synthesized by way of precursor proteins, that each hormone has a specifically related neurophysin and that maturation probably occurs *in granulo* during intra-axonal transport, it seems reasonable to suggest that the precursor for vasopressin may also be the precursor for vasopressin–neurophysin (Sachs *et al.,* 1969; Pickering *et al.,* 1971; Hope and Pickup, 1974). Thus, there may be two prohormones—pro-oxytocin giving rise to oxytocin and oxytocin-neurophysin and provasopressin leading to vasopressin and vasopressin–neurophysin. This would explain the specific biosynthetic association of one neurophysin with vasopressin and one with oxytocin.

E. The Significance of the Third Neurophysin

As we have discussed in Section III, the posterior pituitary glands of most of the species examined contain not two neurophysins but three and, although the third component is usually present in much smaller amounts than the other two, its presence must be accounted for. One must ask if it is associated with a third active peptide (Hope and Pickup, 1974)—even the guinea pig, in which only one major neurophysin has been found, contains a minor component (Watkins and Ellis, 1973). Certainly, other biologically active peptides have been isolated from the gland, such as coherin, which affects gastrointestinal mobility (Goodman and Hiatt, 1972), and the polypeptide with oxytocic activity isolated by Hope and Watkins (1969), but we have suggested an alternative explanation, namely, that the minor neurophysin component is a metabolic product of one of the major ones (Burford and Pickering, 1973; Pickering *et al.*, 1974, 1975).

As can be readily seen in Fig. 9, the time-course for the labeling of the minor component in the rat (NpC) is quite different from that for the two major neurophysins, with the former not becoming appreciably labeled until after the latter have reached their peak labeling. Moreover, all three neurophysins are found within neurosecretory granules (which show the same time-course for labeling as the major neurophysins) (Swann and Pickering, 1974b, 1976) so that a possible interpretation from Fig. 9 is that NpC arises *in granulo* from one of the major components after arrival in the neural lobe. Evidence that this interpretation might be correct came from an observation which, at first sight, was at variance with our original hypothesis for the association of NpA with vasopressin and NpB with oxytocin. Once the major neurophysins in the neural lobe had reached their peak of labeling following intracisternal injection of ^{35}S-labeled cysteine, their radioactivity fell off exponentially and, as shown in Fig. 10a, could be expressed as log-linear regressions. Both NpA and NpB gave good straight lines, but the slopes of these lines were significantly different from each other meaning that the ratio of radioactivity associated with NpA to that associated with NpB increased with time after injection of the isotope. Our first evidence for the association of one neurophysin with one hormone was that this radioactive ratio was equal to 1.5, the vasopressin: oxytocin ratio (Burford *et al.*, 1971a), whereas the comparison of the regression lines showed that this was only true for the first 24 hours after injection and placed considerable strain on the hypothesis. Since the

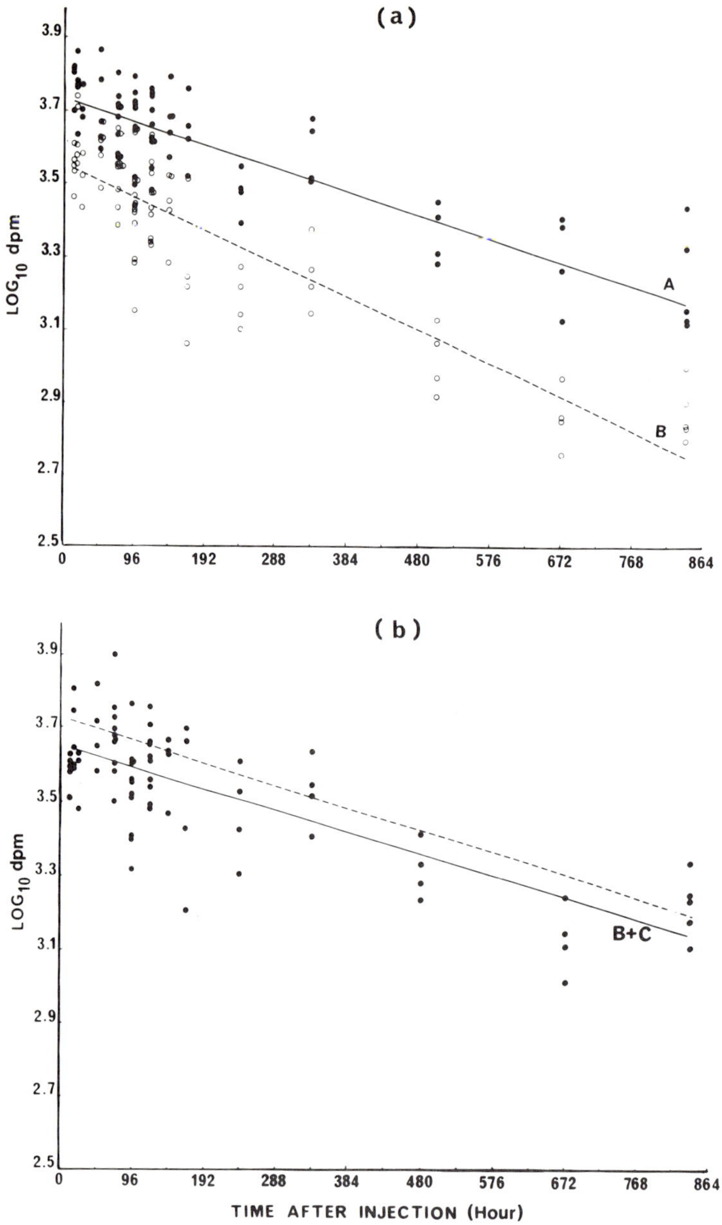

FIG. 10. Decline in radioactivity of the neurophysins in the rat neural lobe after an intracisternal injection of 50 μCi of ^{35}S-labeled cysteine. (a) The major neurophysins A and B. (b) The sum of the radioactivity in neurophysins B and C, with the line for A shown dotted. The points show the results of individual experiments, and the curves are the calculated lines of best fit. Equations of the lines were: $\log N_A = 3.73–6.33 \times 10^{-4}t$; $\log N_B = 3.55–9.40 \times 10^{-4}t$; $\log N_{B+C} = 3.65–6.02 \times 10^{-4}t$. (From Pickering *et al.*, 1975.)

time-course (Fig. 9) suggested that the minor component (NpC) might be arising in the neural lobe, it seemed reasonable to ask whether the faster decline of the radioactivity of NpB (Fig. 10) might be associated with the appearance of label in NpC. Accordingly, for each time interval the sum of the radioactivity in NpB, together with that in NpC was determined, and this was found to give a log-linear regression with a slope that was parallel to the corresponding line for NpA (Fig. 10b). Such a relationship of the sum of NpB and NpC with NpA is more strikingly illustrated in the heterozygous Brattleboro rat (Fig. 11). In this animal, there is more oxytocin than vasopressin in the gland, and, at early times after injection of ^{35}S-labeled cysteine, there is more radioactivity associated with NpB than with NpA. The radioactivity of NpB, however, declines so much faster than that in NpA that the ratio is reversed, although once again, when the sum of NpB and NpC is considered as a single entity, its decline parallels that of NpA (Fig. 11b) (Mallam and Jones, 1974). Thus, these observations are compatible with the suggestion that NpC might arise in the granule from NpB after the NSG have arrived in the neural lobe. North *et al.* (1977) have recently reported that incubation of rNpII (B) with neural lobe extract at pH 4.8 converted it into a component having the electrophoretic properties of rNpIII. Moreover, a similar relationship

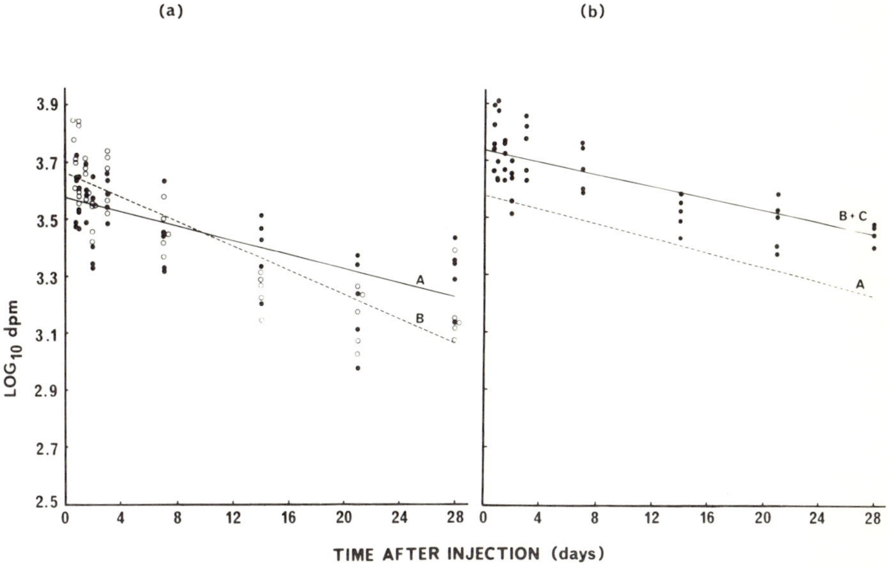

FIG. 11. Decline in radioactivity associated with the neurophysins of the heterozygous Brattleboro rat after an intracisternal injection of 50 μCi of ^{35}S-labeled cysteine. Effect of summating NpB and NpC. (From Pickering *et al.*, 1975.)

seems to exist among the porcine neurophysins, since Wuu and Crumm (1976b) have shown that pNpIII consists of the molecule of pNpI with an additional -Arg-Arg-Ala at the COOH terminus. Thus, if pNpI arises from pNpIII inside the granule, the true porcine vasopressin (pNpIII) is almost identical with its bovine counterpart (bNpII).

The evidence available at present is, thus, compatible with a common biosynthetic origin of each neurohypophyseal hormone and its respective neurophysin as depicted in Fig. 12. This is analogous to the sequence of events that is known to occur in the β-cell of the pancreas where proinsulin is synthesized in a ribosomal system, packaged into granules in the Golgi complex and subsequently "matured" *in granulo* to insulin and C peptide (see Steiner, 1969; Steiner *et al.,* 1973; Grant *et al.,* 1971). Thus, the secretory granules contain a "maturase" enzyme which, we would suggest (Fig. 12), in the oxytocin granules of the rat, continues to digest NpB to give rise to the minor component NpC. In the pig, it would seem that such a continued digestion proceeds more rapidly so that in the gland as removed there is more pNpI than pNpIII.

F. The Nature of the Hormone–Neurophysin Precursor

In spite of considerable effort, no laboratory has yet been able to isolate the precursor or, indeed, to positively identify it with a chromatographic peak or electrophoretic band.* Walter and his co-workers from pulse-chase experiments in both the dog (Walter *et al.,* 1977) and the guinea pig (Mendelson and Walter, 1977) have begun to obtain such evidence of bands that become labeled quickly after a pulse of tracer and then decline as radioactivity begins to appear in neurophysin. Antibodies raised against the rat neurophysins (McPherson and Pickering, 1977) revealed an excess of immunoreactive neurophysinlike material in hypothalamic extracts on the basis of their hormone content, and, hopefully, if this excess represents precursor, these antibodies may be of use in its purification (Pickering and McPherson, 1977).

* Very recently, Gainer and colleagues (1977a,b) have given evidence for just such a precursor in the rat. One hour after an injection of [^{35}S]cysteine into the supraoptic nucleus (SON) a radioactive component with molecular weight about 20,000 could be demonstrated in extracts of the SON. An hour later (i.e., 2 hours postinjection) this was still the major component in SON extracts, but in extracts of the median eminence it was accompanied by another radioactive component with the mobility of neurophysin in the acid–urea–polyacrylamide system which they used. Twenty-four hours after injection, this second component represented almost all of the radioactivity recovered from gels run with extracts of both median eminence and neural lobe. The authors interpret their findings in terms of maturation of a neurophysin precursor during intraaxonal transport much as proposed in Fig. 12.

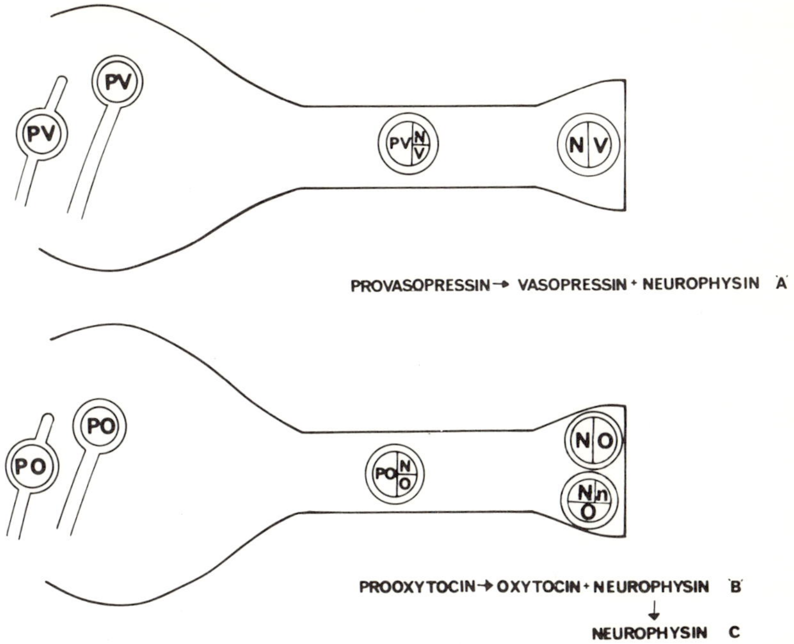

FIG. 12. Hypothetical scheme showing the relationship of neurophysins and hormones in the rat. (From Pickering *et al.,* 1975.)

In view of the evidence linking the hormones and their respective neurophysins to common precursor molecules, it is pertinent to ask what the nature of the linkage in the prohormones is likely to be. Because of the presence of a COOH-terminal glycinamide in all of the neurohypophyseal hormones, it has been assumed hitherto that any linkage between neurophysin and hormone is likely to involve the NH_2-terminal of the hormone, and such a hypothetical scheme has been outlined by Hope and Pickup (1974). However, Smyth (Bradbury *et al.,* 1976) has proposed that the presence of a COOH-terminal amide group in a peptide hormone (e.g., α-MSH) suggests that it may be derived from its prohormone by transamidation. In accordance with this suggestion, Fig. 13 shows the hypothetical structure (or partial structure) for bovine pro-oxytocin in which the hormone is linked to the neurophysin by a glycylalanine bond. It may be pertinent to point out that every neurophysin which has been studied, albeit very few, has an alanine residue at the NH_2 terminal (Wuu *et al.,* 1971; Walter *et al.,* 1971; Capra *et al.,* 1972, 1974), since D. G. Smyth (personal communication) notes that the glycylalanine bond is one of the most susceptible to transamidation.

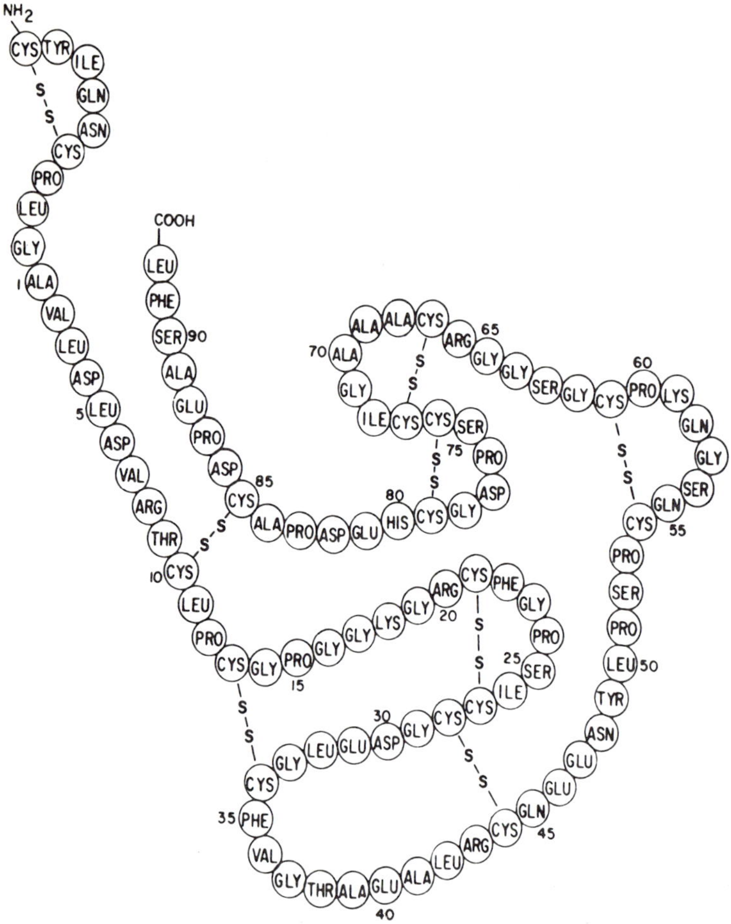

FIG. 13. A speculative suggestion for the structure of the oxytocin precursor (Pro-oxytocin). (After Bradbury *et al.*, 1976, and Schlesinger *et al.*, 1977a.)

VI. Interaction of the Neurophysins with the Neurohypophyseal Hormones

A. NATURE OF THE INTERACTION

The first indication that the van Dyke protein might not contain the oxytocic and vasopressor active moieties in *chemical* linkage came from the observation (Haselbach and Piguet, 1952) that oxytocic activity could be dissociated from a high MW protein by electrodialysis. However, it was the work of R. Acher and his collaborators in Fromageot's laboratory in Paris that first focused attention on the interaction of an "inert" protein (neurophysin) and the nonapeptide hormones (Acher *et al.,* 1955, 1956; Acher and Fromageot, 1957; Chauvet *et al.,* 1960). They showed that, while the biologic activities of the van Dyke protein could not be dissociated as small peptides if the protein were dissolved and dialyzed against water, they were readily dialyzable if the protein were dialyzed against dilute acetic acid. This finding was further amplified by Lindner *et al.* (1959), who showed that when posterior pituitary extracts were chromatographed on the newly available Sephadex at pH 5.9, the biologic activities were almost entirely associated with a high MW protein. When, however, this fraction was rechromatographed on the same column, but at pH 1, the hormonal peptides were well separated from the inactive protein—a finding which was to be of use in the purification of neurohypophyseal hormones from many sources (e.g., Fig. 14).

These observations of the effects of pH on the association–dissociation of neurophysin and the hormones suggested that ionic interaction might be the important bonding for the formation of the complex. When Ginsburg and Ireland (1963, 1964) used the thin film dialysis technique (Craig *et al.,* 1957) to study the binding of the hormones to purified bovine neurophysin at various pH values, they obtained curves (Fig. 15) which could best be interpreted in terms of the interaction of an α-NH_2 group with a side-chain COOH group. Since neither oxytocin nor vasopressin contains a free carboxyl, it was logical to conclude that the binding was between the α-NH_2 of the hormone and a COOH in the neurophysin. Further evidence for this conclusion was published at the same time by Stouffer *et al.* (1963), who showed that a hormone analog lacking an α-NH_2 group, [1-deamino]oxytocin, will not bind to neurophysin; more recently, Hope and Walti (1971) showed that another highly potent analog in which the α-NH_2 was replaced by a hydroxyl, [1-(L-2-hydroxy-3-mercaptopropionic acid)]-oxytocin, was also unable to bind to neurophysin. Changes in H^+ ion equilibria consequent on binding (Breslow *et al.,* 1971) are also in accord with the sharing of a proton between the hormone α-NH_2 group and a COOH group in the protein (Breslow, 1974).

Although electrostatic interaction is a requirement for binding at least at moderate pH, the high specificity of neurophysins for neurohypophyseal hormonelike peptide molecules indicates the presence of constraints additional to the presence of a free α-NH_2 group. In 1966, Breslow and Abrash examined the binding characteristics of a number of analogs of oxytocin. They showed that the relative position of the disulfide bond and the α-NH_2 group is of little importance for binding since [1-hemihomocysteine]-oxytocin bound as well as oxytocin. However, the same workers found that all modifications of the 2 position in oxytocin

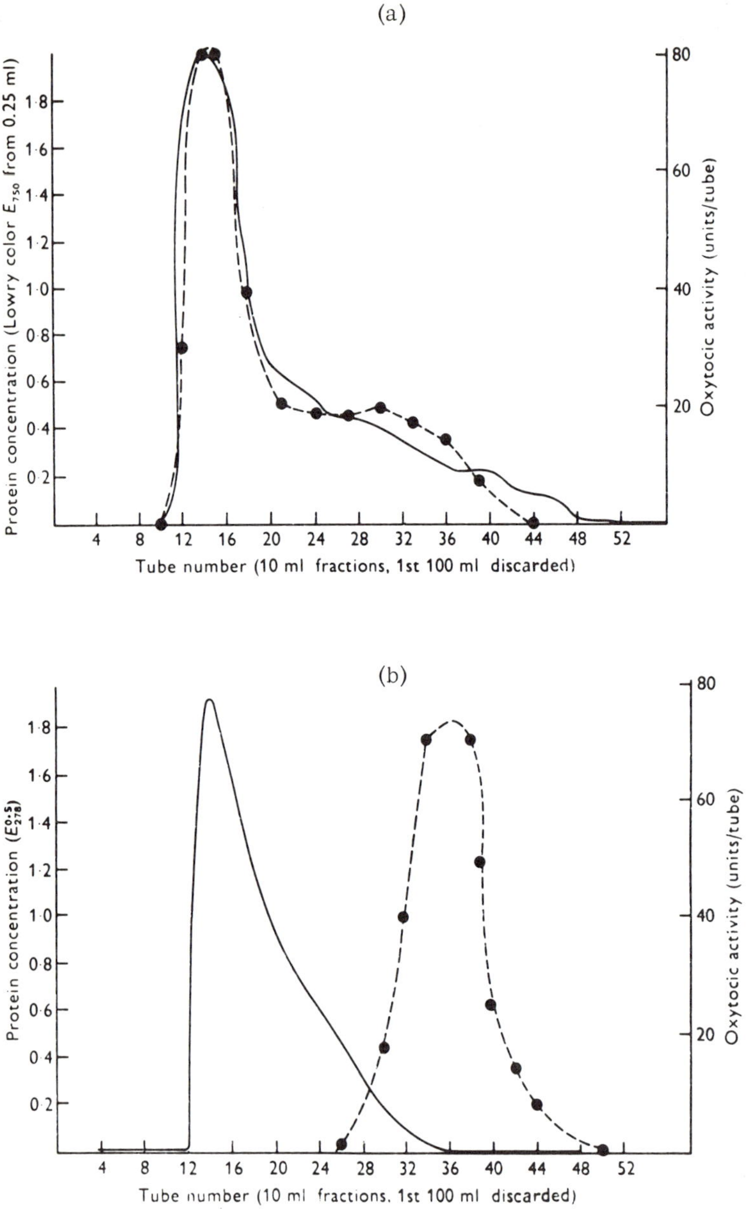

FIG. 14. Use of neurophysin–hormone complex in the isolation of neurohypophyseal hormones. (a) Chromatography of a pituitary extract from cod on Sephadex G-25 at pH 5.8. (b) Rechromatography of the protein peak (tubes 10–20) on the same column as in (a), but after equilibration and elution with 0.05 *M* acetic acid. Note that, at pH 5.8, the hormones chromatographed as a protein complex which was dissociated under acidic conditions. (From Pickering, 1968.)

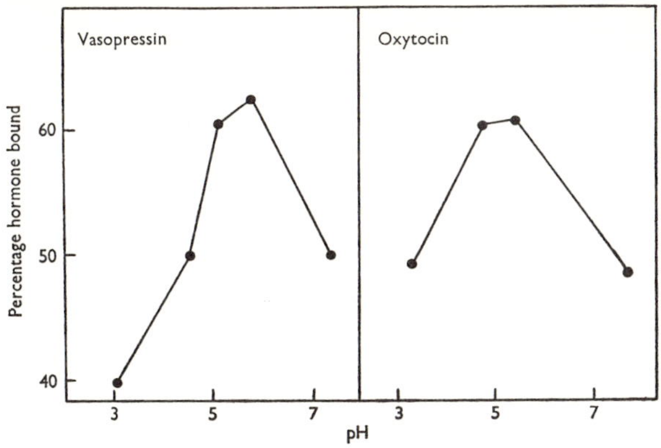

FIG. 15. Effect of pH on the binding of neurophyseal hormones to neurophysin. (From Ginsburg and Ireland, 1964.)

(normally a Tyr residue), except removal of the hydroxyl to give [2-phenylalanine]-oxytocin, led to a virtual abolition of binding, and they concluded that hydrophobic or π–π interactions between position 2 in oxytocin and groups in neurophysin are important for binding. Replacement of the isoleucine residue in position 3 of oxytocin with a glycine also led to loss of binding showing that this residue too was involved in hydrophobic bonding. Breslow and her colleagues (Breslow *et al.*, 1973; Breslow, 1975) have confirmed and extended those observations by the use of di- and tripeptide analogs of the three residues at the amino terminal of oxytocin. Summarizing these results, it is clear that the most important contributions to binding are residues 1 and 2 of the hormones, since dipeptide analogs to these residues (e.g., Met-TyrNH_2) bind to neurophysin with a free energy change equal to almost 60% of that seen during hormone binding (Breslow, 1975). In addition, Breslow's (1975) data indicate that there is cooperativity between residues 1 and 2 during binding. Other physicochemical studies also indicate an interaction of residues 1, 2, and 3 of the hormone during binding and that the aromatic residues in positions 2 and 3 of vasopressin enter a hydrophobic environment when this hormone binds (Furth and Hope, 1970; Griffin *et al.*, 1973; Balram *et al.*, 1973). In other words, as Furth and Hope (1970) put it, the hormone molecule appears to enter the protein "head first."

Each of the bovine neurophysin molecules has a single tyrosine residue present in position 49 (Walter *et al.*, 1971; North *et al.*, 1975). Furth and Hope (1970) nitrated this residue in bovine NpII and showed that this did not affect the hormone-binding ability of the protein. The use of this reporter group has shown that, when binding occurs, nitro-Tyr^{49} becomes fully ionized (even at pH 6.2), consistent with the approach of a positively charged group (Furth and Hope, 1970). Later studies (Breslow and Weiss, 1972) indicate that this effect more probably comes about from the neutralization of a neighboring negatively charged carboxyl (by the α-NH_2 of the hormone), rather than a direct effect of the positive group on the tyrosyl residue. Alternatively, Griffin *et al.* (1973), who also studied the effects of model peptides on spectral changes suggested that the effects in the ionization of Tyr^{49} might come about from its removal to a less hydrophobic environment consequent to binding. Breslow (1975) has suggested a model (Fig. 16) which summarizes present ideas about changes at the binding site and is not very different from a similar model proposed by Griffin *et al.* (1973).

B. Number of Binding Sites

The first attempts to determine the capacity of neurophysin for the binding of hormonal peptides (i.e., number of binding sites per molecule) were made by Ginsburg and his associates (Ginsburg and Ireland, 1965; Ginsburg *et al.*, 1966). In these early experiments, the unbound hormone was measured by bioassay after equilibrium dialysis so that the range of free hormone concentrations amenable to study was necessarily limited. For this reason, the values obtained for estimates of the maximum binding capacity of neurophysin were subject to a fair degree of error. Nevertheless, these early findings suggested that bovine neurophysin could bind 3.6 moles of arginine vasopressin (AVP), and porcine neurophysin could bind 4 moles of lysine vasopressin (LVP) per 25,000 gm protein. In the same experiments, the capacity for oxytocin binding was estimated as 7 and 14 moles/25,000 gm for the bovine and porcine protein, respectively. The authors realized that their inability to work with an extended range of hormone concentrations was liable to give falsely high estimates, and, in a later paper, where ^{14}C-labeled vasopressin allowed lower concentrations to be used, the binding capacity of porcine neurophysin for LVP was revised to 1 mole/12,000 gm protein (Ginsburg and Thomas, 1969).

It is now generally agreed that bovine NpI and bovine NpII have one binding site for oxytocin per monomer of 10,000 MW (Breslow and Abrash, 1966; Breslow and Walter, 1972; Camier *et al.*, 1973). However, there is no such accord with regard to the capacity of bovine Np for LVP. On the one hand, the American workers (see Breslow, 1974, 1975) find a single binding site for LVP which, on the basis of competition experiments, would appear to be identical with the oxytocin-binding site, while, on the other hand, the French group (Camier *et al.*, 1973; Cohen *et al.*, 1975) find two thermodynamically equivalent sites for LVP. Moreover, in their hands, competitive studies between LVP and oxytocin have suggested that the binding sites for the two hormones are not identical but that there is partial overlap of one of the LVP sites with the oxytocin site (Camier *et al.,* 1973). By examining the changes in proton equilibrium and circular dichroism occurring during the binding of LVP to bovine NpII with different proportions of peptide and protein, Breslow *et al.,* (1973) excluded the possibility of two thermodynamically equivalent sites but allowed the possibility of a second site with a much lower affinity than the first. Interestingly, Pliška and Sachs (1974) concluded that the interaction of LVP and bovine NpII involved the participation of two populations of binding sites one of them with an association constant for LVP of about $10^7 M^{-1}$ and the other about $10^4 M^{-1}$. Moreover, the relative proportions of these two populations of sites varied with the neurophysin concentration although this ratio remained constant if the neurophysin were coupled to agarose beads. These effects would be explained by the tendency of neurophysin to polymerize (Burford *et al.,* 1969, 1971b) and resolve the difference between the apparent association constant of 10^6–$10^7 M^{-1}$ found by Ginsburg's group (Burford *et al.,* 1969, 1971b) at low neurophysin concentrations and that of 2.5×10^4 found (Breslow and Abrash, 1966;

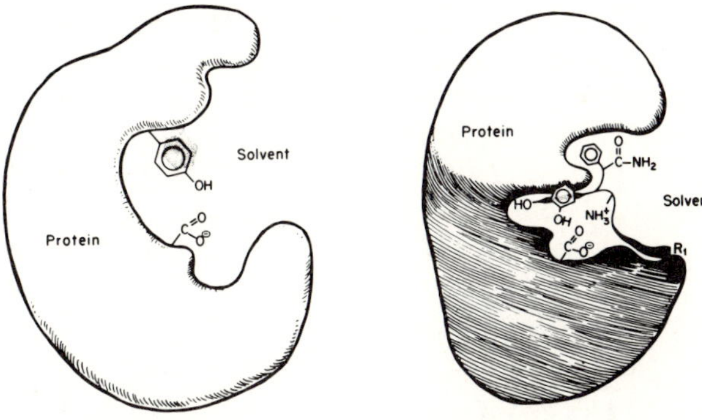

FIG. 16. Possible model for the binding of a tripeptide to bovine NpII. In the absence of peptide, Tyr_{49} of NpII is stacked with a phenylalanine residue and moderately close to the side chain carboxyl that forms part of the peptide-binding site. In the presence of peptide, a conformational change occurs in the protein. Stacking between Tyr_{49} and the protein phenylalanine is lost (for simplicity, the phenylalanine is not shown, since its location relative to bound peptide cannot be inferred from the data), and Tyr_{49} is now located close to Tyr_2 of the peptide, with an angle between the plane of the two rings intermediate between 0° and 90°. The shaded region of the complex can be envisioned as bending behind the unshaded region, so that Tyr_{49} is fully exposed to solvent, but Tyr_2 is enclosed in a hydrophobic pocket, in part shielded by Tyr_{49}. The salt bridge between the α-NH_2 of the peptide and protein carboxyl is also shown as protected from solvent by neighboring apolar interactions. Interactions between the side chain of residue $1(R_1)$ and residue 3 (here shown as $PheNH_2$) are regarded as apolar, but not very sterically restricted. (From Breslow, 1975.)

Breslow and Walter, 1972; Camier *et al.,* 1973) at much higher concentrations (Pliška and Sachs, 1974).

However, this still does not resolve the difference between Breslow and co-workers and Cohen and associates about the number of binding sites for LVP and NpII. The data from each laboratory allow no interpretation other than the one drawn. This being so, the difference must arise either from some difference in experimental technique, which seems unlikely, or from some difference in the preparation of bovine Np used. The latter suggestion seems more likely and could easily be tested by an exchange of samples between the two laboratories. There are good reasons for expecting that such differences may occur, since Pliška and his colleagues (Pliška *et al.,* 1974; Pliška and Meyer-Grass, 1975) have shown that "native" neurophysins, isolated from NSG by mild conditions, have different binding characteristics from the usual preparations of the proteins that have been extracted with strong acids, often from acetone-dried pituitaries. Their "native" neurophysins, which contained hexosamine and fatty acids, and, thus, might be analogous to the lipoproteinlike neurophysin described by Mylroie and Koenig (1971), showed evidence of a single population of binding sites with high affinity (K_{ass} about $10^7 M^{-1}$) and could be converted into "conventional neurophysins," with overall K_{ass} about $10^4 M^{-1}$, by treatment with either strong acid or strong alkali (Pliška and Meyer-Grass, 1975). Thus, it might be that the French and American neurophysin preparations might differ in their degree of nativeness. In this context, it is interesting that, when "French" bovine NpII which showed two equivalent binding sites was nitrated, the resulting nitroneurophysin (see Fig. 17) had only one binding site per molecule (Cohen *et al.,* 1975).

Very recently, Cohen and his colleagues (Nicolas *et al.,* 1976) have

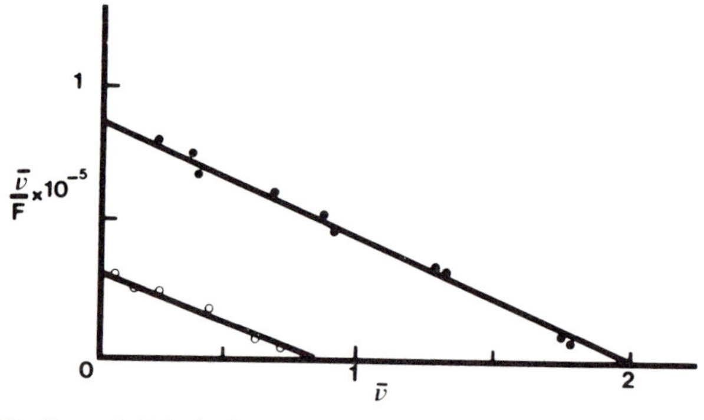

FIG. 17. Binding of [8-lysine]-vasopressin to native (○) and nitrated (●) bovine neurophysin I. (From Cohen *et al.,* 1975.)

offered an explanation of the discrepancies. They interpret their results to suggest that neurophysin exists as a monomer with 2 binding sites/10,000 daltons in equilibrium with a dimer having 2 sites/20,000 daltons with the other two sites masked during aggregation. Furthermore, their results suggest that oxytocin displaces the equilibrium in favor of the dimer so that study of its binding parameters suggests 1 site/10,000 while, on the other hand, lysine vasopressin at high concentrations binds preferentially to the monomeric neurophysin and, thus, shifts the equilibrium toward this form, and gives a figure of 2 sites/10,000. Low concentrations of vasopressin bind preferentially to dimeric neurophysin giving 1 site/10,000 and, hence, the discrepancy between laboratories described above could be explained in terms of the concentrations of ligand used in each case. Moreover, it was possible to induce oxytocin to bind to 2 sites/10,000 by the addition of a high concentration of LiCl, although this did not appear to affect the monomer $\rightleftharpoons$ dimer equilibrium (Nicolas *et al.,* 1976).

C. Effects of Ca^{2+} on the Hormone–Neurophysin Interaction

The first indication that calcium ions might affect hormone–neurophysin interaction came from the observation of Smith and Thorn (1965) that crude bovine neurophysin decreased the elution volume of AVP during chromatography on Sephadex G-25 and that this effect was abolished by Ca^{2+}. Several reports from Ginsburg's group also pointed to an inhibition of the binding reaction by Ca^{2+}. As measured by equilibrium dialysis, $10^{-6} M$ calcium completely inhibited the binding of oxytocin by crude porcine neurophysin (Ginsburg *et al.,* 1966). Elution-analysis of gel filtration experiments (Burford *et al.,* 1969) and sedimentation studies (Burford *et al.,* 1971b) suggested that Ca^{2+} interfered with the polymerization equilibria of the protein and stabilized a dimeric form, irrespective of protein concentration. On the other hand, numerous workers have been unable to find any effects of Ca^{2+} on hormone–neurophysin binding reactions (Breslow, 1970; Breslow *et al.,* 1971; Camier *et al.,* 1973; Pliška and Sachs, 1974), and one wonders once again whether these differences are due to small differences (degree of nativeness) among the protein preparations used. It would be interesting to know, in this context, whether Ca^{2+} influences hormone binding by the "native" neurophysin preparation of Pliška and Meyer-Grass (1975).

VII. Measurement of Neurophysins

Neurophysin will produce antibodies in the rabbit quite readily, and a number of radioimmunoassay systems have been developed, using bovine

(Legros *et al.,* 1969; Martin *et al.,* 1972; Robinson *et al.,* 1971a) porcine (Uttenthal *et al.,* 1971; Cheng and Friesen, 1971b; Pickup *et al.,* 1973), and human (Cheng and Friesen, 1973; Robinson and Zimmerman, 1973; Robinson, 1974, 1975a) proteins. In many cases, antibodies have been used that will easily distinguish between the two major proteins of a given species so that they may be measured individually.

Much of the experimental work on the physiology of the hypothalamo-neurohypophyseal system has been done with the laboratory rat, and, in many cases, confusion has come about by the use of immunoassays developed for neurophysins of other species. An ideal radioimmunoassay should be conducted with an antibody raised against the substance to be measured (e.g., rat neurophysin) and with the same substance as a reference standard. Heterologous radioimmunoassays (i.e., those where the antigen is not identical to the substance being measured) should also be used with the substance being measured as reference standard. This is mandatory if absolute amounts rather than relative changes in concentrations are to be measured, although in cases when a stoichiometric cross-reaction has been shown throughout the concentration range used in the assay, it is permissible, though not desirable, to use a heterologous protein as a reference preparation.

Now that purified rat neurophysins are available, together with some specific or partially specific antibodies to the individual proteins (Pickering *et al.,* 1975; McPherson and Pickering, 1975), it should be possible to quantitate the changes in the release of the separate neurophysins from rat glands under various experimental conditions. An alternative approach to this problem has been described by Sunde and Sokol (1975) who have used polyacrylamide gel electrophoresis to quantitate the amounts of the neurophysins in rat glands by measuring the intensity of the blue bands after staining the gels with amido black. Although the caveats about the nature of the reference standard still apply, the errors are likely to be smaller in the more chemical determinations than in ones relying on immuno-cross-reactivity. However, the polyacrylamide gel method carries with it other errors, since it assumes that the stained bands in the neurophysin region contain only neurophysin.

VIII. Does Neurophysin Have a Systemic Biologic Role?

A. Metabolic Effects

The occurrence of biologic activity in neurophysin preparations was recognized at an early stage of neurophysin research. Many neurophysin preparations, and, especially the porcine ones, have been endowed with a variety of biologic activities including lipolytic, hyperglycemic, hypocalcemic, and serum amino acid lowering effects.

Over a number of years, Rudman and co-workers have demonstrated biologic activity in successive preparations from porcine pituitaries. These peptides, H, L, and, finally, 7 D6, which were, in fact, increasingly purer preparations of pNpI, were shown to have a lipolytic action in rabbit adipose tissue and to cause hyperglycemia and hypoaminoacidemia in the rabbit and monkey (Rudman *et al.,* 1970). At the same time, Astwood and colleagues were able to isolate a major constituent from porcine posterior pituitaries and showed that their "peptide II" was the same as Rudman's 7D6 peptide. Peptide II had lipolytic activity in rabbit adipose tissue, but not in that of the rat.

More recently, Trygstad *et al.* (1975) have purified the three neurophysins from human glands and have shown that these peptides have biologic activity. All three (hNpI, hNpII, and hNpIII) had significant lipolytic effects in human and rabbit fat but had no such activity in rat or mouse tissue. The hypocalcemic effect observed earlier in rabbits, using porcine neurophysin preparations (Friesen, 1964), was also seen when the human neurophysins were injected i.v. into rabbits or human subjects. A prolonged hyperglycemic effect, apparently unrelated to the lipolytic action, was also observed, but only with hNpIII. All three human neurophysins were able to cause a lowering of blood amino acid levels in both man and rabbit.

Recent studies by Rudman *et al.* (1975) have cast a great deal of light onto the whole subject of neurophysin-associated biologic activity. They prepared a bovine preparation analogous to the 7D6 porcine preparation. This peptide (bNpI) showed both lipolytic and melanotropic activities. However bNpI, bNpII, and hNpI prepared by preparative PAGE in Wal-

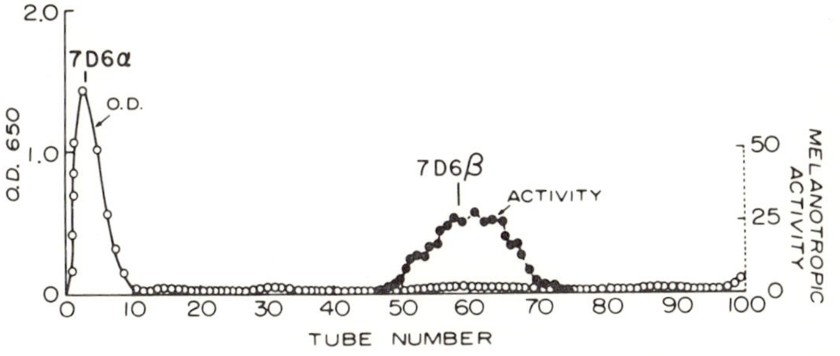

FIG. 18. Separation of a melanotropic peptide from a preparation of a neurophysinlike protein (Rudman's D76) by countercurrent distribution. The protein (100 mg) was distributed in the system 1-butanol/0.1 *M* NH_4HCO_3. (From Rudman *et al.*, 1975.)

ter's laboratory were devoid of any such biologic activity despite the fact that, for example, the different preparations of bNpI were indistinguishable in terms of amino acid analysis and electrophoretic mobility. These findings suggested that the biologic activities of the various neurophysins were due to a contaminant. Rudman *et al.* (1975) went on to show that countercurrent distribution of their bovine 7D6 preparation (bNpI) separated biologically inactive bNpI from a small MW peptide with melanotropic and lipolytic activity (see Fig. 18). This small peptide had an MW of a few thousand and appears to resemble in both amino acid composition, electrophoretic mobility, and biologic activity a peptide "11F" found in many extrahypophyseal tissues.

B. Renal Effects

Other investigators have demonstrated that neurophysin preparations have natriuretic actions, and Robinson *et al.* (1975) showed that bNpI but not bNpII was able to cause natriuresis by decreasing proximal tubular reabsorption of Na^+. Similar experiments carried out with bNpI samples obtained by preparative PAGE, although indistinguishable immunologically, did not produce a consistent natriuretic response, and it was suggested that the initial preparations of bNpI, which were purified by ion-exchange chromatography alone, were contaminated with a non-neurophysin substance responsible for the natriuretic action.

Cort *et al.* (1975) have investigated the binding of small peptides with natriuretic activity to porcine neurophysin. Crude van Dyke protein prepared in the classical manner is natriuretic. Gel filtration of the crude preparation at low pH, not only dissociates oxytocin and vasopressin from the neurophysin peak, but it also separates the natriuretic activity. Electrophoresis of the small peptide fraction revealed that the natriuretic activity was associated with a region which had an R_f different from those of oxytocin and vasopressin (Cort *et al.*, 1975). Amino acid analysis of this peptide showed a molar ratio of amino acids that could be expected for α-MSH or ACTH 1-13. Although the intrinsic natriuretic activity of such peptides is small, they could attain a significant natriuretic role by potentiating the natriuretic actions of AVP. It is not known whether these peptides are derived from the pars intermedia tissue, included during gland collection, or whether they occur naturally within the neural lobe.

The above investigations suggest that biologic activities assigned to the neurophysins are, in all probability, due to the presence of contaminating, biologically active peptides that remain associated with the inert neurophysins even after multiple chromatographic steps. This fact is highlighted by the observations from Walter's laboratory, where it was noted that, during sequence studies with a bovine neurophysin I preparation, purified by ion exchange chromatography, proteolysis yielded a hexapeptide that had no relationship at all to the rest of the neurophysin sequence (see Discussion after North *et al.,* 1975). Perhaps, in the case of the neurophysins, the lack of real biologic activity in the molecule has enabled the presence of contaminants to be uncovered. However, only careful interlaboratory collaboration will allow the inertness of pure neurophysins to be established or refuted.

Apparently, then, we are without an extraneurohypophyseal biologic role for neurophysins, even though in terms of weight, it is the major secretory product of the hypothalamo-neurohypophyseal system. The significance of the presence of immunologically reactive material in hypophyseal portal blood (Zimmerman *et al.,* 1973), and in tissues such as anterior pituitary, kidney, uterus, and striated muscle (Ginsburg and Jayasena, 1968; Legros *et al.,* 1975a remains to be established.

IX. Speculations on the Evolution of Neurophysin

The sequence of amino acids in the neurophysin molecule shows several areas of similarity and apparent repetition. Taking bNpI as an example: within the two regions of the molecule from positions 12 to 31 and from 60 to 77, there are several stretches of amino acids which are the same in both. Oddly enough, the two seven-membered rings, Cys^{21}–Cys^{27} and Cys^{67}–Cys^{73}, which are closed by disulfide bridges and which occur one in each area, show little homology within the rings, even though five of the six surrounding residues are identical. These rings and surrounding regions may represent disulfide bonds preserved after a reduplication process (see below). Similarly, two regions with homologous sequences within them can be seen in the sequences of other neurophysins (Fig. 19). The length of chain between residues 32 and 59 does not appear to be duplicated, and Capra and Walter (1975) speculate that if the neurophysin monomer carries only one hormone-binding site, then this site is likely to be situated in an unduplicated region. It is interesting that this stretch of the molecule not only contains an invariant polar region (43–49) enclosing the bonds (Leu^{42}/Arg^{43} and Arg^{43}/Cys^{44}), which are most susceptible to proteolysis, but also contains Tyr^{49} which has been implicated in the binding reaction (see Section VI,A). Capra and Walter also point out that, if the neurophysin molecule were to possess two binding sites, as some data suggest, these would be expected to reside in the duplicated region of the molecule.

How can these intramolecular structural similarities have arisen? One

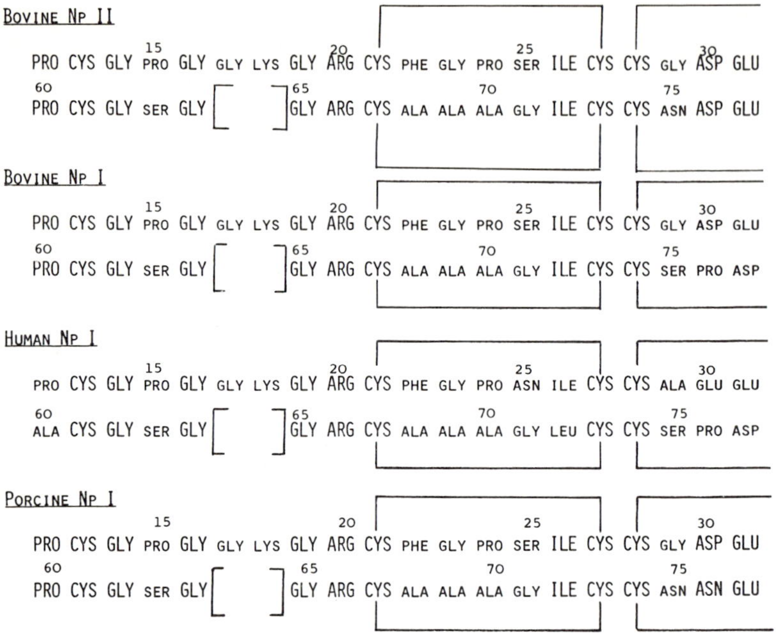

FIG. 19. Demonstration of sequence duplication within the neurophysin molecule. The sequences have been interrupted (see brackets) to show maximal homology. (After Capra and Walter, 1975.)

possible explanation is that, at some time during evolution of the neurophysins, gene duplication and fusion have occurred. One can envisage that a primitive gene coding for a 50–60 residue ancestral molecule underwent gene duplication with partial fusion to yield a gene now coding for a protein of about 10,000 daltons MW, containing regions of similar sequences within the molecule. Apparently even a disulfide bridge ring (the seven-membered Cys^{21}–Cys^{27} and Cys^{67}–Cys^{73}) present in the ancestral protein was maintained in the duplication process, and the amino acid arrangement around the disulfide bond reproduced. There is now considerable evidence supporting the process of gene duplication and fusion as a major process in the evolution of a number of protein molecules—the IgG and IgM immunoglobulins (Edelman *et al.,* 1969; Putnam *et al.,* 1973), bacterial ferredoxins and growth hormone, prolactin, and placental lactogen (Niall *et al.,* 1971). Later on, possibly during the emergence of the primitive vertebrates, the duplicated but fused gene must have undergone a further, complete, duplication resulting in the presence of two neurophysin genes, and, hence, two neurophysins in each species.

It is interesting that precisely this kind of gene duplication has been proposed to account for the phylogenetic distribution of the neurohypophyseal hormones themselves (see Pickering and Heller, 1969). Only one hormone (arginine vasotocin) has been detected in the present day cyclostomes and hagfishes, while the neurohypophyses of more advanced vertebrates contain two. If, as seems likely, (see Section V,D) each hormone shares a common biosynthetic precursor with its neurophysin, only one such protein should be present in the cyclostomes. It will be interesting to study the phylogeny of the neurophysins and to compare the chemistry of these molecules with those of the proteins present in the neurosecretory granules of other animals—e.g., the sulfur-rich protein in the granules of insects (Steel and Morris, 1975).

References

Abel, J. J. (1924). *Bull. Johns Hopkins Hosp.* **35,** 305–328.
Abel, J. J. (1930). *J. Pharmacol. Exp. Ther.* **40,** 139–169.
Acher, R. (1958). *Proc. Int. Symp. Neurosecretion 2nd, 1957* pp. 71–78.
Acher, R. (1976). *Biochimie* **58,** 895–911.
Acher, R., and Fromageot, C. (1957). *In* "The Neurohypophysis" (H. Heller, ed.), pp. 39–50. Butterworth, London.
Acher, R., Manoussos, G., and Olivry, G. (1955). *Biochim. Biophys. Acta* **16,** 155–156.
Acher, R., Chauvet, J., and Olivry, G. (1956). *Biochim. Biophys. Acta* **22,** 421–427.
Acher, R., Light, A., and du Vigneaud, V. (1958). *J. Biol. Chem.* **233,** 116–120.
Albers, R. W., and Brightman, M. W. (1959). *J. Neurochem.* **3,** 269–276.
Balram, P., Bothner-By, A. A., and Breslow, E. (1973). *Biochemistry* **12,** 4695–4704.
Barer, R., Heller, H., and Lederis, K. (1963). *Proc. R. Soc. London, Ser. B* **158,** 388–416.
Bargmann, W. (1949). *Z. Zellforsch. Mikrosk. Anat.* **34,** 610–634.
Block, R. J., and van Dyke, H. B. (1952). *Arch. Biochem. Biophys.* **36,** 1–4.
Bradbury, A. F., Smythe, D. G., and Snell, C. R. (1976). *Ciba Found. Symp.* **41,** 61–75.
Breslow, E. (1970). *Proc. Natl. Acad. Sci. U.S.A.* **67,** 439–495.
Breslow, E. (1974). *Adv. Enzymol.* **40,** 271–333.
Breslow, E. (1975). *Ann. N.Y. Acad. Sci.* **248,** 423–441.
Breslow, E., and Abrash, L. (1966). *Proc. Natl. Acad. Sci. U.S.A.* **56,** 640–646.
Breslow, E., and Walter, R. (1972). *Mol. Pharmacol.* **8,** 75–81.
Breslow, E., and Weiss, J. (1972). *Biochemistry* **11,** 3474–3482.
Breslow, E., Aanning, H. L., Abrash, L., and Schmir, M. (1971). *J. Biol. Chem.* **246,** 5179–5188.
Breslow, E., Weis, J., and Menendez-Botet, C. J. (1973). *Biochemistry* **12,** 4644–4653.
Burford, G. D., and Pickering, B. T. (1971). *J. Endocrinol.* **51,** xiv–xv.
Burford, G. D., and Pickering, B. T. (1972). *Biochem. J.* **128,** 941–944.
Burford, G. D., and Pickering, B. T. (1973). *Biochem. J.* **136,** 1047–1052.
Burford, G. D., Ginsburg, M., and Thomas, P. J. (1969). *J. Physiol. (London)* **205,** 635–646.
Burford, G. D., Jones, C. W., and Pickering, B. T. (1971a). *Biochem. J.* **124,** 809–813.
Burford, G. D., Ginsburg, M., and Thomas, P. J. (1971b). *Biochim. Biophys. Acta* **229,** 730–738.

Camier, M., Alazard, R., Cohen, P., Pradelles, P., Morgat, J. C., and Fromageot, P. (1973). *Eur. J. Biochem.* **32,** 207–214.

Capra, J. D., and Walter, R. (1975). *Ann. N.Y. Acad. Sci.* **248,** 397–407.

Capra, J. D., Kehoe, J. M., Kotelchuck, D., Walter, R., and Breslow, E. (1972). *Proc. Natl. Acad. Sci. U.S.A.* **69,** 431–434.

Capra, J. D., Cheng, K. W., Friesen, H. G., North, W. G., and Walter, R. (1974). *FEBS Lett.* **46,** 71–74.

Chauvet, J., Lenci, M. T., and Acher, R. (1960). *Biochim. Biophys. Acta* **38,** 266–272.

Chauvet, M. T., Chauvet, J., and Acher, R. (1975a). *FEBS Lett.* **52,** 212–215.

Chauvet, M. T., Chauvet, J., and Acher, R. (1975b). *FEBS Lett.* **58,** 234–237.

Chauvet, M. T., Chauvet, J., and Acher, R. (1976). *Eur. J. Biochem.* **69,** 475–485.

Cheng, K. W., and Friesen, H. G. (1971a). *J. Biol. Chem.* **246,** 7656–7665.

Cheng, K. W., and Friesen, H. G. (1971b). *Endocrinology* **88,** 608–619.

Cheng, K. W., and Friesen, H. G. (1972). *J. Clin. Endocrinol. Metab.* **34,** 165–176.

Cheng, K. W., and Friesen, H. G. (1973). *J. Clin. Endocrinol.* **36,** 553–560.

Chrétien, M., and Gilardeau, C. (1973). *Acta Endocrinol. (Copenhagen)* **74,** 226–236.

Cohen, P., Camier, M., Wolff, J., Alazard, R., Cohen, J. S., and Griffin, J. H. (1975). *Ann. N.Y. Acad. Sci.* **248,** 463–479.

Cort, J. H., Sedláková, E., Kluh, I., and Mulder, J. H. (1975). *Ann. N.Y. Acad. Sci.* **248,** 336–344.

Coy, D. H., and Wuu, T. C. (1971). *Anal. Biochem.* **44,** 174–181.

Coy, D. H., and Wuu, T. C. (1972). *Biochim. Biophys. Acta* **263,** 125–132.

Craig, L. C., King, T. P., and Stracher, A. (1957). *J. Am. Chem. Soc.* **79,** 3729–3737.

Cross, B. A., Dyball, R. E. J., Dyer, R. G., Jones, C. W., Lincoln, D. W., Morris, J. F. and Pickering, B. T. (1975). *Recent Progr. Hormone Res.,* **31,** 243–294.

Dale, H. H. (1906). *J. Physiol. (London)* **34,** 163–206.

Dale, H. H. (1909). *Biochem. J.* **4,** 427–447.

Dean, C. R., and Hope, D. B. (1967). *Biochem. J.* **104,** 1082–1088.

Dean, C. R., and Hope, D. B. (1968). *Biochem. J.* **106,** 565–573.

Dean, C. R., Hollenberg, M. D., and Hope, D. B. (1967). *Biochem. J.* **104,** 8C–10C.

Dean, C. R., Hope, D. B., and Kažić, T. (1968a). *Br. J. Pharmacol.* **34,** 192P–193P.

Dean, C. R., Hope, D. B., and Kažić, T. (1968b). *Br. J. Pharmacol.* **34,** 193–194.

Dudley, H. W. (1919). *J. Pharmacol. Exp. Ther.* **14,** 295–312.

Dudley, H. W. (1923). *J. Pharmacol. Exp. Ther.* **21,** 103–122.

Edelman, G. M., Cunningham, B. A., Gall, W. E., Gottlieb, P. D., Rutishauser, U., and Wuxdal, M. J. (1969). *Proc. Natl. Acad. Sci. U.S.A.* **63,** 78–85.

Farini, F. (1913). *Gazz. Osp. Clin.* **34,** 1135–1139.

Foss, I., Sletten, K., and Trygstad, O. (1973). *FEBS Lett.* **30,** 151–156.

Frankland, B. T. B., Hollenberg, M. D., Hope, D. B., and Schacter, B. A. (1966). *Br. J. Pharmacol. Chemother.* **26,** 502–510.

Friesen, H. G. (1964). *Metab. Clin. Exp.* **13,** 1214–1229.

Friesen, H. G., and Astwood, E. B. (1967). *Endocrinology* **80,** 278–287.

Furth, A. J., and Hope, D. B. (1970). *Biochem. J.* **116,** 545–553.

Gainer, H., Sarne, Y., and Brownstein, M. J. (1977a). *Science* **195,** 1354–1356.

Gainer, H., Sarne, Y., and Brownstein, M. J. (1977b). *J. Cell Biol.* **73,** 366–381.

Ginsburg, M. (1964). *Proc. Int. Pharmacol. Meet., 2nd, 1963* Vol. 10, pp. 87–97.

Ginsburg, M. (1968). *Handb. Exp. Pharmacol.* **23,** 286–371.

Ginsburg, M., and Ireland, M. (1963). *J. Physiol. (London)* **169,** 15–16.

Ginsburg, M., and Ireland, M. (1964). *J. Endocrinol.* **30,** 131–145.

Ginsburg, M., and Ireland, M. (1965). *J. Endocrinol.* **32,** 187–198.

Ginsburg, M., and Ireland, M. (1966). *J. Endocrinol.* **35,** 289–298.

Ginsburg, M., and Jayasena, K. (1968). *J. Physiol. (London)* **197,** 65–76.

Ginsburg, M., and Thomas, P. J. (1969). *J. Physiol. (London)* **201,** 181–199.

Ginsburg, M., Jayasena, K., and Thomas, P. J. (1966). *J. Physiol. (London)* **184,** 387–401.

Goodman, I., and Hiatt, R. B. (1972). *Science* **178,** 419–421.

Grant, P. T., Coombe, T. L., Thomas, N. W., and Sargent, J. R. (1971). *Mem. Soc. Endocrinol.* **19,** 481–495.

Griffin, J. H., Alazard, R., and Cohen, P. (1973). *J. Biol. Chem.* **248,** 7975–7978.

Haselbach, C. H., and Piguet, A. R. (1952). *Helv. Chim. Acta* **35,** 2131–2135.

Hild, W. (1951). *Virchows Arch. Pathol. Anat. Physiol.* **319,** 526–546.

Hild, W., and Zetler, G. (1953a). *Pfluegers Arch. Gesamte Physiol. Menschen Tiere* **257,** 169–201.

Hild, W., and Zetler, G. (1953b). *Z. Exp. Med.* **120,** 236–243.

Hollenberg, M. D., and Hope, D. B. (1967). *Biochem. J.* **104,** 122–127.

Hollenberg, M. D., and Hope, D. B. (1968). *Biochem. J.* **106,** 557–564.

Holwerda, D. A. (1972). *Eur. J. Biochem.* **28,** 334–339.

Hope, D. B., and Pickup, J. C. (1974). *Handb. Physiol. Sect. 7: Endocrinol.* **4,** 173–189.

Hope, D. B., and Walti, M. (1971). *Biochem. J.* **125,** 909–911.

Hope, D. B., and Watkins, W. B. (1969). *Br. J. Pharmacol.* **37,** 533P–535P.

Hvas, S., and Thorn, N. A. (1973). *Acta Endocrinol. (Copenhagen)* **74,** 209–214.

Jones, C. W., and Pickering, B. T. (1970). *J. Physiol. (London)* **208,** 73P–74P.

Jones, C. W., and Pickering, B. T. (1972). *J. Physiol. (London)* **227,** 553–564.

Jones, C. W., and Swann, R. W. (1974). *J. Endocrinol.* **63,** 53P–54P.

Jones, C. W., and Swann, R. W. (1975). *J. Physiol. (London)* **245,** 45P.

Jongkind, J. F. (1972). *Prog. Brain Res.* **38,** 59–67.

Kamm, O., Aldrich, T. B., Grote, I. W., Rowe, L. W., and Bugbee, E. P. (1928). *J. Am. Chem. Soc.* **50,** 533–601.

Koenig, H. (1974). *Adv. Cytopharmacol.* **2,** 273–301.

Koenig, H., and Mylroie, R. (1975). *Ann. N.Y. Acad. Sci.* **248,** 218–234.

LaBella, F. S., Reiffenstein, R. J., and Beaulieu, G. (1963). *Arch. Biochem. Biophys.* **100,** 399–408.

LaBella, F. S., Shin, S. H., Vivian, S. R., and Dular, R. (1971). *Mem. Soc. Endocrinol.* **19,** 293–312.

Lederis, K., and Heller, H. (1960). *Acta Endocrinol. (Copenhagen) Suppl.* **51,** 115–116.

Lederis, K., and Jayasena, K. (1970). *Int. Encyclo. Pharmacol. Ther. Sect.* **41,** 111–154.

Legros, J. J., and Louis, F. (1974). *Neuroendocrinology* **13,** 371–375.

Legros, J. J., Franchimont, P., and Hendrick, J. C. (1969). *C. R. Soc. Biol. Ses Fil.* **163,** 2773–2777.

Legros, J. J., Hendrick, J. C., and Franchimont, P. (1970). *C. R. Soc. Biol. Ses. Fil.* **164,** 2389–2395.

Legros, J. J., Stewart, U., Nordmann, J. J., Dreifuss, J. J., and Franchimont, P. (1971). *C. R. Soc. Biol. Ses Fil.* **165,** 2443–2447.

Legros, J. J., Reynaert, R., and Peeters, G. (1974). *J. Endocrinol.* **60,** 327–332.

Legros, J. J., Louis, F., Grötschel-Stewart, U., and Franchimont, P. (1975a) *Ann. N.Y. Acad. Sci.* **248,** 157–171.

Legros, J. J., Reynaert, R., and Peeters, G. (1975b). *J. Endocrinol.* **67,** 297–302.

Lindner, E. B., Elmqvist, A., and Porath, J. (1959). *Nature (London)* **184,** 1565–1566.

MacArthur, C. G. (1931). *Science* **73,** 448.

McNeilly, A. S., Legros, J. J., and Forsling, M. L. (1972). *J. Endocrinol.* **52,** 209–210.

McPherson, M. A., and Pickering, B. T. (1975). *J. Endocrinol.* **67,** 43P–44P.

McPherson, M. A., and Pickering, B. T. (1977). *J. Endocrinol.* In Press.

Mallam, J. B., and Jones, C. W. (1974). *Gen. Comp. Endocrinol.* **22,** 337.

Martin, M. J., Chard, T., and Landon, J. (1972). *J. Endocrinol.* **52,** 481–495.

Matthews, E. K., Legros, J. J., Grau, J. D., Nordmann, J. J., and Dreifuss, J. J. (1973). *Nature (London), New Biol.* **241,** 86–88.

Mendelson, I. S., and Walter, R. (1977). *In* "Hypothalamic Hormones," (W. Voelter, and D. Gupta, eds.). Verlag Chemie; Weinheim (in press).

Morris, J. F. (1976). *J. Endocrinol.* **68,** 209–224.

Morris, J. F., and Cannata, M. A. (1973). *J. Endocrinol.* **57,** 517–529.

Mylroie, R., and Koenig, H. (1971). *J. Histochem. Cytochem.* **19,** 738–746.

Niall, H. D., Hogan, M. L., Sauer, R., Rosenblum, I. Y., and Greenwood, R. C. (1971). *Proc. Natl. Acad. Sci. U.S.A.* **68,** 866–869.

Nicolas, P., Camier, M., Dessen, P., and Cohen, P. (1976). *J. Biol. Chem.* **251,** 3965–3971.

Nordmann, J. J., Dreifuss, J. J., and Legros, J. J. (1971). *Experientia* **27,** 1344–1345.

Norström, A. (1974). *In* "Neurosecretion—The Final Neuroendocrine Pathway" (F. G. W. Knowles and L. Vollrath, eds.), pp. 86–93. Springer-Verlag, Berlin and New York.

Norström, A. (1975). *Ann. N.Y. Acad. Sci.* **248,** 46–63.

Norström, A., and Sjöstrand, J. (1971). *J. Neurochem.* **18,** 2007–2016.

North, W. G., and Valtin, H. (1977). *Anal. Biochem.* **78,** 436–450.

North, W. G., Walter, R., Schlesinger, D. H., Breslow, E., and Capra, J. D. (1975). *Ann. N.Y. Acad. Sci.* **248,** 408–422.

North, W. G., Valtin, H., Morris, J. F., and La Rochelle, F. T. (1977). *Endocrinology* **101,** 110–118.

Oliver, G., and Schafer, E. A. (1895). *J. Physiol. (London)* **18,** 277–279.

Ott, I., and Scott, J. C. (1910). *Proc. Soc. Exp. Biol. Med.* **8,** 48–49.

Palay, S. L. (1957). *In* "Ultrastructure and Cellular Chemistry of Neural Tissue" (H. Waelsch, ed.), pp. 31–49. Harper (Hoeber), New York.

Paton, D. N., and Watson, A. (1912). *J. Physiol. (London)* **44,** 413–424.

Pickering, B. T. (1968). *J. Endocrinol.* **42,** 143–152.

Pickering, B. T., and Heller, H. (1969). *J. Endocrinol.* **45,** 597–606.

Pickering, B. T., and McPherson, M. A. (1977). *In* "Neurohypophysial Hormones" (A. M. Moses and M. Miller, eds.) (in press).

Pickering, B. T., Jones, C. W., and Burford, G. D. (1971). *Ciba Found. Study Group* **39,** 58–74.

Pickering, B. T., Jones, C. W., and Burford, G. D. (1974). *In* "Neurosecretion—The Final Common Pathway" (F. G. W. Knowles and L. Vollrath, eds.), pp. 72–85. Springer-Verlag, Berlin and New York.

Pickering, B. T., Jones, C. W., Burford, G. D., McPherson, M., Swann, R. W., Heap, P. F., and Morris, J. F. (1975). *Ann. N.Y. Acad. Sci.* **248,** 15–35.

Pickup, J. C., Johnston, C. I., Nakamura, S., Uttenthal, L. O., and Hope, D. B. (1973). *Biochem. J.* **132,** 361–371.

Pliška, V., and Meyer-Grass, M. (1975). *Ann. N.Y. Acad. Sci.* **248,** 235–245.

Pliška, V., and Sachs, H. (1974). *Eur. J. Biochem.* **41,** 229–239.

Pliška, V., McKelvy, J. F., and Sachs, H. (1972). *Eur. J. Biochem.* **28,** 110–115.

Pliška, V., Meyer-Grass, M., and Sunde, D. (1974). *In* "Neurosecretion—The Final Neuroendocrine Pathway" (F. G. W. Knowles and L. Vollrath, eds.), p. 319. Springer-Verlag, Berlin and New York.

Putnam, F. W., Florent, G., Paul, C., Shinoda, T., and Shimizu, A. (1973). *Science* **182,** 287–291.

Rauch, R., Hollenberg, M. D., and Hope, D. B. (1969). *Biochem. J.* **115,** 473–479.

Rennels, M. L. (1966). *Endocrinology* **78,** 659–660.

Robinson, A. G. (1974). *J. Clin. Invest.* **54,** 209–212.

Robinson, A. G. (1975a). *J. Clin. Invest.* **55,** 360–367.

Robinson, A. G. (1975b). *Ann. N.Y. Acad. Sci.* **248,** 246–256.

Robinson, A. G., and Zimmerman E. A. (1973). *J. Clin. Invest.* **52,** 1260–1267.

Robinson, A. G., Zimmerman, E. A., and Engleman, E. G. (1971a). *Metab. Clin. Exp.* **20,** 1138–1147.

Robinson, A. G., Zimmerman, E. A., and Frantz, A. G. (1971b). *Metab., Clin. Exp.* **20,** 1148–1155.

Robinson, A. G., Michelis, M. F., Warms, P. C., and Davis, B. B. (1975). *Ann. N.Y. Acad. Sci.* **248,** 317–323.

Rosenfield, M. (1940). *Bull. Johns Hopkins Hosp.* **66,** 398–403.

Rudman, D., Del Rio, A. E., Garcia, L. A., Barrett, J., Howard, C. H., Walker, W., and Moore, G. (1970). *Biochemistry* **9,** 99–108.

Rudman, D., Chawla, R. K., Khatra, B. S., and Yodaiken, R. E. (1975). *Ann. N.Y. Acad. Sci.* **248,** 324–335.

Sachs, H. (1969). *Adv. Enzymol.* **32,** 327–372.

Sachs, H. (1970). *Int. Encyclop. Pharmacol. Ther., Sect.* **41,** 155–171.

Sachs, H. (1971). *Mem. Soc. Endocrinol.* **19,** 965–973.

Sachs, H., and Takabatake, Y. (1964). *Endocrinology* **75,** 943–948.

Sachs, H., Fawcett, C. P., Takabatake, Y., and Portanova, R. (1969). *Recent Prog. Horm. Res.* **25,** 447–491.

Sachs, H., Goodman, R., Osinchak, J., and McKelvy, J. (1971a). *Proc. Natl. Acad. Sci. U.S.A.* **68,** 2782–2786.

Sachs, H., Saito, S., and Sunde, D. (1971b). *Mem. Soc. Endocrinol.* **19,** 325–336.

Sachs, H., Pearson, D., and Nureddin, A. (1975). *Ann. N.Y. Acad. Sci.* **248,** 36–45.

Sawyer, W. H. (1961). *Pharmacol. Rev.* **13,** 225–277.

Scharrer, E., and Scharrer, B. (1954). *In* "Handbuch der mikroskopischen Anatomie des Menschen" (W. von Möllendorff and W. von Bargmann, eds.), Vol. 6, No. 5, pp. 953–1066. Springer: Berlin.

Schlesinger, D. H., Frangione, B., and Walter, R. (1972). *Proc. Natl. Acad. Sci. U.S.A.* **69,** 3350–3354.

Schlesinger, D. H., Ernst, M., Nicholas, A., Watkins, W. B., and Walter, R. (1975). *FEBS Lett.* **57,** 55–59.

Schlesinger, D. H., Ernst, M., Audhya, T. K., and Walter, R. (1977a). *Massachusetts General Hospital Research Symposium.* In press.

Schlesinger, D. H., Pickering, B. T., Watkins, W. B., Peek, J. C., Moore, L. G., Audhya, T. K., and Walter, R. (1977b). *FEBS Lett.* In press.

Sloper, J. C. (1954). *J. Anat.* **88,** 576–577.

Sloper, J. C. (1955). *J. Anat.* **89,** 301–316.

Sloper, J. C. (1958). *Int. Rev. Cytol.* **7,** 337–389.

Smith, M. W., and Thorn, N. A. (1965). *J. Endocrinol.* **32,** 141–151.

Steel, C. G. H., and Morris, G. P. (1975). *Gen. Comp. Endocrinol.* **26,** 517–524.

Steiner, D. F. (1969). *N. Engl. J. Med.* **280,** 1106–1113.

Steiner, D. F., Rubenstein, A. H., Peterson, J. D., Kemmler, W., and Tager, H. S. (1973). *In* "Endocrinology" (R. O. Scow, F. J. G. Ebling, and I. W. Henderson, eds.), pp. 561–566. Elsevier, New York.

Stouffer, J. E., Hope, D. B., and du Vigneaud, V. (1963). *In* "Perspectives in Biology" (C. F. Cori, *et al.*, eds.), pp. 75–80. Elsevier, Amsterdam.

Sunde, D. A., and Sokol, H. W. (1975). *Ann. N.Y. Acad. Sci.* **248,** 345–364.

Swann, R. W., and Pickering, B. T. (1974a). *J. Endocrinol.* **61,** lvi–lvii.

Swann, R. W., and Pickering, B. T. (1974b). *J. Endocrinol.* **63,** 51P–52P.

Swann, R. W., and Pickering, B. T. (1976). *J. Endocrinol.* **68,** 95–108.

Takabatake, Y., and Sachs, H. (1964). *Endocrinology* **75,** 934–942.

Trygstad, O., Foss, I., and Sletten, K. (1975). *Ann. N.Y. Acad. Sci.* **248,** 304–316.
Uttenthal, L. O., and Hope, D. B. (1970). *Biochem. J.* **116,** 899–909.
Uttenthal, L. O., Livett, B. G., and Hope, D. B. (1971). *Philos. Trans. R. Soc. London, Ser. B* **261,** 380–381.
Valtin, H., Sawyer, W. H., and Sokol, H. W. (1965). *Endocrinology* **77,** 701–706.
van Dyke, H. B., Chow, B. F., Greep, R. O., and Rothen, A. (1942). *J. Pharmacol. Exp. Ther.* **74,** 190–209.
Vogt, M. (1953). *Br. J. Pharmacol. Chemother.* **8,** 193–196.
von den Velden, R. (1913). *Berl. Klin. Wochenschr.* **50,** 2083–2086.
Walter, R., ed. (1975). "Neurophysins: Carriers of Peptide Hormones," Ann. N.Y. Acad. Sci. No. 248. N.Y. Acad. Sci., New York.
Walter, R., and Audhya, T. K. (1977). *In* "Neurohypophysial Hormones" (A. M. Moses and M. Miller, eds.) (in press).
Walter, R., Schlesinger, D. H., Schwartz, I. L., and Capra, J. D. (1971). *Biochem. Biophys. Res. Commun.* **44,** 293–298.
Walter, R., Audhya, T. K., Schlesinger, D. H., Shin, S., Saito, S., and Sachs, H. (1977). *Endocrinology* **100,** 162–174.
Watkins, W. B. (1971). *J. Endocrinol.* **51,** 595–596.
Watkins, W. B. (1972a). *J. Endocrinol.* **55,** 577–589.
Watkins, W. B. (1972b). *Biochem. J.* **126,** 759–760.
Watkins, W. B. (1973). *J. Endocrinol.* **59,** 17–29.
Watkins, W. B., and Ellis, H. K. (1973). *J. Endocrinol.* **59,** 31–41.
Weinstein, H., Malamed, S., and Sachs, H. (1961). *Biochim. Biophys. Acta* **50,** 386–889.
Weiss, P. (1944). *Anat. Rec.* **88,** 464.
Weiss, P. (1968). "Dynamics of Development: Experiments and Inferences." Academic Press, New York.
Wuu, T. C., and Crumm, S. E. (1973). *Proc. Int. Congr. Biochem., 9th 1973* Abstract Db9, p. 453.
Wuu, T. C., and Crumm, S. F. (1976a). *Biochem. Biophys. Res. Commun.* **68,** 634–639.
Wuu, T. C., and Crumm, S. F. (1976b). *J. Biol. Chem.* **251,** 2735–2739.
Wuu, T. C., and Saffran, M. (1969a). *Protein Polypeptide Horm., Proc. Int. Symp., 1968* Excerpta Med. Found., Int. Congr. Ser. No. 161, pp. 477–481.
Wuu, T. C., and Saffran, M. (1969b). *J. Biol. Chem.* **244,** 482–490.
Wuu, T. C., Crumm, S., and Saffran, M. (1971). *J. Biol. Chem.* **246,** 6043–6063.
Zimmerman, E. A., Carmel, P. W., Husain, M. K., Ferin, M., Tannenbaum, M., and Robinson, A. G. (1973). *Science* **182,** 925–927.

5

Separation Methods and Arne Tiselius

JERKER PORATH

Having been asked to present my personal opinion about the research on separation methods at the Institute of Biochemistry in Uppsala, I have chosen to emphasize particularly the impact which the personality and work of Arne Tiselius have had on the development of research here (Tiselius, 1968; Keckwich and Pedersen, 1974). As the founder of the Institute, he began a tradition of biochemical methodology, which is still very much alive among those of us who were his pupils and followers. Tiselius, in turn, built upon the foundation in colloid and polymer chemistry which was laid by his teacher Theodor Svedberg (Fig. 1, b) during the three first decades of this century. From Svedberg, he inherited his interest for methodology and his appreciation for precision in physical measurements.

Arne Wilhelm Kaurin Tiselius, together with Theodor Svedberg, made some of the most outstanding contributions to Swedish scientific research during this century. He was born August 10, 1902, in Stockholm. On the paternal side, he belonged to a family with a traditional link to the exact sciences. Both his father and grandfather were mathematicians. His mother, Rosa Kaurin, was born in Norway of Scottish descent. After his father's death in 1906, the family moved to Gothenburg, where Arne Tiselius was to spend the years of his childhood and youth.

Arne Tiselius obtained his schooling at the Göteborgs Högre Realläroverk where, under the tutelage of his chemistry teacher, Ludvig Jönsson, he was stimulated to pursue a deeper understanding of the discipline. The written reports of the pupil's first experiments are still in existence. They describe a number of investigations in the chemistry of mercury salt complexes; the results are presented in a remarkably clear and penetrating manner. Characteristic of these reports are the sharp formula-

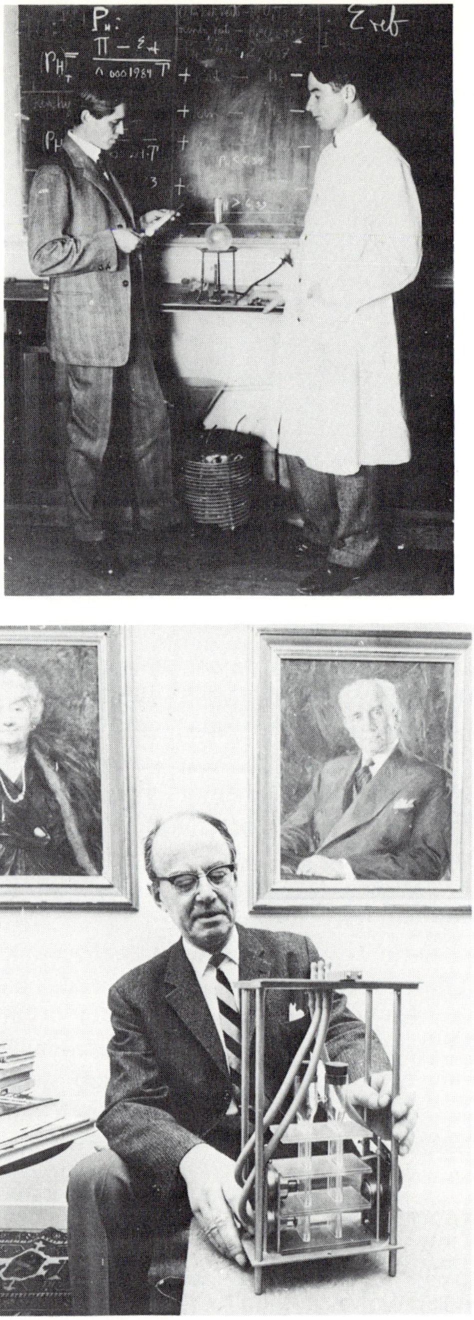

FIG. 1. (a) Arne Tiselius, as a young student, with his teacher, Theodor Svedberg, in the Institute of Chemistry, 1926. (b) Arne Tiselius, at the time of his retirement, behind his electrophoresis cell constructed in 1937.

tion of the problem at hand, the precision in the observations, the notations of all deviation from the expected results, the summary of results, along with subsequent conclusions that form the basis for new series of experiments. These methodical basic principles, so maturely formulated and followed already when Tiselius was 18, are, henceforth, significant for Arne Tiselius' *modus operandi*, in the laboratory as well as in the library.

As a 19-year-old youth, Arne Tiselius arrived in Uppsala, Sweden's learned city par excellence and the site of its oldest university, which at the time was merely a small country town. From above the entrance to the chemistry building, three giants, sculptured in stone, were looking down upon the young student: Wilhelm Scheele, Torbern Bergman, and Jöns Jacob Berzelius. A fourth giant within Swedish chemistry was very much alive and active inside the building. Theodor Svedberg remained a youth of boundless vitality all through his life, which remarkedly enough ended the same year as that of our young student of 1921 vintage.

Arne Tiselius passed his courses in mathematics, physics, and chemistry and was awarded his first academic degree at the age of 22. He had thus been exposed to, and acquired, a good knowledge of the so called "dry and wet analysis," the former of which had been introduced by Berzelius and remained a tradition at the Institute as late as the early 1940's, when I was a chemistry freshman. The inorganic chemistry had a strong position in Uppsala, as well as in other parts of Sweden; historically, it had sprung out of the country's metallurgical pursuits and was brought up to the ranks of an art through Berzelius and his pupils.

Swedish chemistry does, however, have roots also within other domains. Physical chemistry had made a leap forward through the work of Svante Arrhenius, who at the beginning of Tiselius' academic career, was more often stationed by the telescope than at the microscope or the lab bench. Theodor Svedberg did, however, lead with an indefatigable enthusiasm a hard-working group of students and collaborators, nearly all of whom, in due time, became luminaries within Swedish science and industry. This group was joined in 1925 by Arne Tiselius, who became Svedberg's personal assistant—an immense honor that was accompanied by a heavy responsibility for the young student.

Tiselius published his first work with Svedberg in 1926 under the title "A New Method for Determination of Mobility of Proteins" (Svedberg and Tiselius, 1926). Of great importance for the focusing of his interest on cataphoresis (electrophoresis) became the task of preparing a survey of the subject for Abderhalden's "Handbuch der Biologischen Arbeitsmethoden"—a task which Svedberg had handed over to his young and promising collaborator (Tiselius, 1927). A deeper knowledge of colloid chemistry was developed when Tiselius was asked to assist in editing a new and expanded edition of Svedberg's well-known monograph on colloid chemistry (New York, 1928). His first publication under sole authorship in 1926 constitutes a theoretical study on the thermodynamical properties of colloids, such as could be measured at the time by means of ultracentrifugal analysis. Six years later, he performed an in-depth study on the influence of electrolytes upon sedimentation rates of colloidal particles (Tiselius, 1932). These early works demonstrate Tiselius' interest and capacity to tackle theoretical physical chemical problems, an attribute which he retained through his entire life, even though his later work mostly concentrated upon practical refinements of already existing methods, along with the development of new procedures and techniques in applied chemistry.

Tiselius' inaugural dissertation "On the Moving Boundary Method of Studying the Electrophoresis of Proteins," dated 1930, represents his largest piece of work. In this monograph, he developed the theory for a moving boundary from the equation of Kohlrausch and Weber, whereby special attention is focused on the spreading or sharpening of the boundary layer (with changes in field strength). In order to perform mobility determinations with the highest possible accuracy, while keeping boundary disturbances to a minimum, he constructed a new apparatus (Fig. 2). A U tube of quartz was used as a separation chamber. This chamber was in contact with an electrode vessel equipped with reversible Ag/AgCl electrodes, and the entire construction is such that heating was strongly reduced in comparison with the earlier apparatus. The separation chamber was photographed using UV light with suitable filters, and the migration of the boundary was measured microphotometrically from the photography. Tiselius prepared a number of proteins with then conventional techniques, such as precipitation and dialysis, and studied them in his apparatus under a variety of conditions. This piece of work can be characterized as a masterful Swedish doctoral thesis in physical chemistry, in which he carefully studied and commented on the sources of error, while suggesting ways to suppress or avoid them. He was awarded the highest possible grade—a prerequisite for a further career at the University, where he immediately obtained a time-limited docentship. His outlook on the future was not bright, however, and his remaining papers and notebooks from this period are marked by great anguish. No chair in biochemistry existed. Svedberg was still young; the only remaining possibility was to attempt to qualify for a chair in inorganic chemistry. With this goal in mind, Tiselius took up studies on diffusion and adsorption in zeolites. During one summer, he collected zeolite specimens on the Faroe Islands and organized equipment for physicochemical studies of his crystals. The experiments were carried out partly by himself and partly in

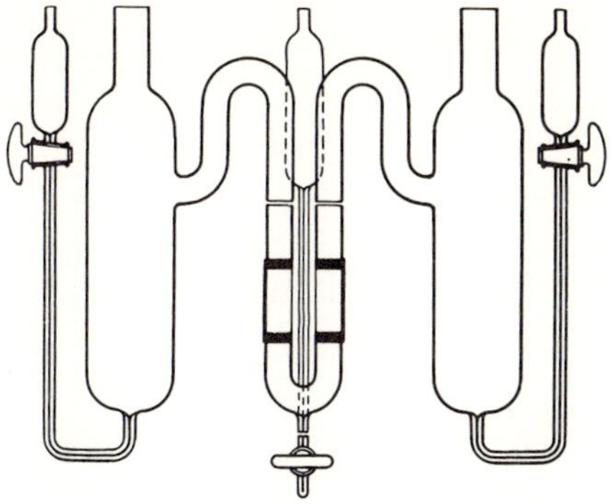

FIG. 2. The electrophoresis apparatus used by Tiselius in his doctoral work.

collaboration with a young student, Sven Brohult (later to become president of the Swedish Academy for Engineering Sciences). Water regained at different temperatures was followed with a sensitive balance; simultaneously, they studied the diffusion of vapor into crystals which had been relieved of their lattice water at a given partial pressure. These crystals were placed in a particularly sensitive evacuation chamber, and, by means of a polarization microscope, they were able to observe double refraction and extinction angles, thereby relating their change to the degree of hydration. Tiselius determined the diffusion constants by inserting the recorded data into the diffusion equation after integration, according to Boltzmann. He also demonstrated that ammonia at low pressures adsorbs to analcite, according to the Langmuir isotherms, and the rates of adsorption were determined at different pressures (Tiselius, 1936). One part of these latter studies were carried out at Princeton University, where Tiselius spent the years 1934–1935 as a Rockefeller scholar under the aegis of Hugh S. Taylor at the Frick Chemical Laboratory. There is no doubt that these studies on the zeolites form a very important background for his later work on adsorption analysis.

In spite of all efforts, Tiselius failed to reach his goal, i.e., the long-sought-for professorship, although he was declared to be very competent. His stay in America did, however, have some very beneficial consequences through the close relations he established with such scientists as J. Northrop, W. Stanley, L. Michaelis, M. Heidelberger, and M. L. Anson. These colleagues inspired him to once again take up the work on electrophoresis, and, after his return to Uppsala, he constructed a new apparatus for this purpose (Fig. 3).

In a 1937 paper titled "A New Apparatus for Electrophoretic Analysis of Colloidal Mixtures," Tiselius (1937a) investigated certain limiting factors and adapted the dimensions of the apparatus to optimal performance.

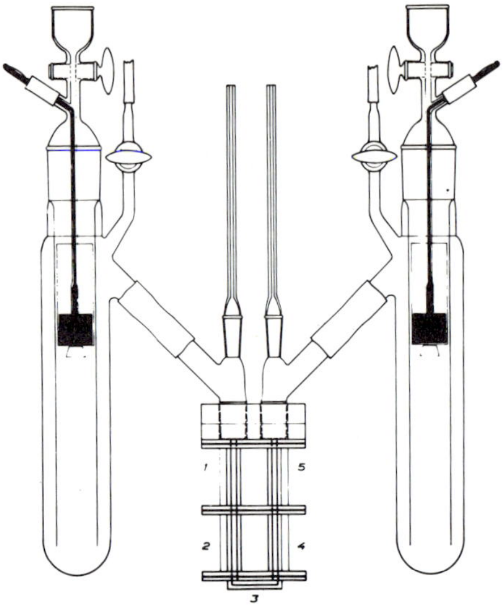

FIG. 3. The electrophoresis cell of the Tiselius apparatus of 1937.

He calculated the minimum volumes for the electrode vessels necessary to avoid ionic migration from the electrode solution and into the separation chamber. The latter was constructed out of planely ground quartz and had a parallellepiped form. It was divided into two sections that could slide on top of each other in order to create a sharp boundary, and to allow removal of the material in each section by pipetting after the electrophoretic separation. The displacement was carried out pneumatically to prevent vibration and the resulting disturbances of the boundaries.

To reduce convection, the apparatus was lowered into a refrigerated bath, the temperature of which was kept close to the density maximum of water (around +4°), since the thermal convection depends on $d\pi/dT$ (π being the density of water at temperature T), which is 0 at this temperature. By so doing, Tiselius increased the wattage by a factor of 10, which enabled him to perform very efficient separations. The best separations were, however, obtained when two substances, A and B, had the same direction of migration and, often, substantial mobilities. This implied that a very long separation chamber might be needed, which would substantially complicate the measurements in the chamber sections. Instead, he let the liquid in the cells stream with a velocity which was adjusted to partly counteract the electrophoretic displacement. By this method, he contained the boundaries for substances of nearly identical mobilities within the separation chamber for extended periods of time and, thereby, increased the resolving power.

In order to observe the boundaries during a run, Tiselius used the Töpler schlieren method supplemented by a refraction method, which he had earlier proposed and later developed together with Ole Lamm, another one of Svedberg's collaborators. The improved electrophoresis apparatus became an Aladdin's lamp with which chemists around the world were able to penetrate and evaluate the protein content of living matter. A number of important contributions were made in Tiselius' own laboratory in Uppsala during the last 3 years of the 1930's. These contributions, which even today seem impressive, were made under the direction of Tiselius himself, along with Kabat, Horsfall, Svensson (Rilbe), Seibert, and Blix. Some of the more important discoveries are worth mentioning. Tiselius himself was able to demonstrate in the first papers (1937b, c) how the plasma proteins can be separated by an electric field into distinct families characterized by differences in electrophoretic mobility. The component which migrates most rapidly in the field under neutral or weakly alkaline conditions is identified as serum albumin. The different classes of globulins are given names from the Greek alphabet, with α as the most mobile, followed by the β and γ fractions. Together with Kabat, Tiselius was able to demonstrate that, in horse antipneumococcus serum, a new component emerges which lies between the β- and γ-globulin fractions, and that this component is identical with the antibodies directed against the bacteria (Tiselius and Kabat, 1938). Through studies of rabbit antisera, they were also able to show that antibodies are associated with proteins in the γ-globulin region. The impact of these findings on immunology and immunochemistry can hardly be overemphasized. For Tiselius personally and for chemistry in Uppsala, these contacts with the leading immunochemists of the time, in particular with Heidelberger and Kabat, were of the utmost importance. From Tiselius' remaining notes, it is evident that the problem of antibody structure and function was a dominant research theme during his whole active career. The gradual shift in emphasis from electrophoresis to chromatography, which took place in the early 1940's, is the result of his growing recognition of the limitations inherent in electrophoresis as a means for further separation and purification of the γ-globulins. Another field in which the inadequacies became evident was the isolation of peptides from protein hydrolyzates, which by necessity had to precede a determination of protein primary structure.

Before leaving Tiselius' applications in the area of moving boundary electrophoresis which span the years 1936–1940, and which could be considered to mark the highlight of his scientific career, we ought to recognize his contributions in the field of lipoprotein chemistry made together with Blix and Svensson, his fractionation of naturally antigenic extracts, exemplified by the purification of tuberculin performed together with

Seibert, and, above all, his work with Horsfall on the dissociation and reconstitution of hemocyanin (Tiselius and Horsfall, 1939). With the perspective of time, it seems to me that these hemocyanin studies are the most important. They constitute a continuation of the studies by Svedberg and Eriksson-Quensel on the pH stability of the hemocyanins. These latter authors used the ultracentrifuge as an analytical instrument, whereas Tiselius and Horsfall made use of the new electrophoresis apparatus. The hemocyanins were prepared from blood originating from *Helix pomatia* and *Helix nemoralis,* and their electrophoretic mobilities were determined. After dissociation in a borate buffer of pH 8.5, the different hemocyanins were reassociated in the original buffer (a phosphate buffer, pH 6.8 and ionic strength 0.1). One studies such "reassociates," both for individual proteins and for mixtures of dissociation products from the different species. The authors found reassociation to take place spontaneously, giving rise to a small amount of synthetic hybrid molecules out of the mixtures from different species. The composition of the product of association indicates a strong preferential formation of the original molecular assembly, and a certain blocking of the formation of hybrids. The latter effects depend on the phylogenetic distance between the species. The authors were fully aware of the principle of this work for the understanding of the assembly of complex protein molecules, today referred to as quaternary structure. On the other hand, Tiselius and Horsfall drew parallels between the reassociation of the monomer mixtures and the formation of mixed crystals between substances of similar chemical structure.

The detailed work on protein characterization, which was made possible by the new technique, would not have been so successful without refinement of the optical tools. In Uppsala, Lamm, Svensson (Rilbe), and Philpot (visiting research fellow from England) contributed substantially to the *mise en point* of the electrophoresis technique. Contributions of equal importance were, however, made in other quarters, above all by Longsworth at The Rockefeller Institute in New York. In the field of theory, great contributions were made by Svensson (Rilbe) in Uppsala and by Dole, Longsworth, and Alberty in the United States. The theoretical investigations aided in suppressing, and in certain cases, in eliminating the sources of error,particularly the so-called boundary anomalies. Tiselius always stressed the gentleness of the electrophoresis method toward the material under investigation, with its implications for the discovery of complexes between proteins or between a protein and other substances, which might be of importance for the biologic function.

A weakening interest for the electrophoresis method was paralleled by an increasing interest in chromatography. Around 1940, he began his studies on the adsorption by active charcoal of amino acids, peptides, and carbohydrates. He constructed special equipment for the procedure—a "filter" and an interferometer—in which he was assisted by his young and promising pupil, Stig Claesson, who later became the successor of Theodor Svedberg as professor of Physical Chemistry in Uppsala. Tiselius (1940, 1943) classified chromatography in three categories: elution analysis, frontal analysis, and displacement analysis. He preferred the name adsorption analysis, rather than chromatography, since the substances need not be colored in order to be detected interferometrically. He soon found that elution analysis was not generally applicable, and, accordingly, his efforts were turned toward the development of the displacement analysis, both in theory and practice. He often used isotherm diagrams to describe the chromatographic processes, and his interpretations of isotherms were based on the adsorption theory of Langmuir. The practical results of this work must be considered as rather limited and are completely overshadowed by the partition chromatography that was developed contemporarily in England by Martin and Synge. This pair of scientists developed personal contacts with Tiselius that were beneficial for the continued work both in England and in Uppsala.

Tiselius originally envisioned that the adsorption behavior in charcoal chromatography was governed by rather simple rules. When he came to realize that this was not the case, he tried to adjust the technique through a number of ingenious tricks. Since there were no sharp borderlines between the different zones in displacement chromatography, he introduced "carrier substances" (Tiselius and Hagdahl, 1950) to increase the separation between the various components of the sample. Unfortunately, carrier displacement chromatography did not live up to his original expectations. This could be explained from the shape of the carrier isotherms, which often crossed those of the test substances, thereby confounding the starkly simple and elegant theory on which the modified displacement analysis was based.

These failures forced Tiselius to think along other lines. I am inclined to regard the gradient elution technique as his most important contribution to the practical application of chromatography. It was first developed in the late 1940's and early 1950's in collaboration with R. J. P. Williams and R. Alm (Alm *et al.*, 1952), then visiting scientists in Uppsala, and L. Hagdahl, who was Tiselius' technician. Long before this work was published, Tiselius had been comtemplating the use of gradient techniques. In his remaining notebooks, I have found plans for an automatic device for "gradient chromatography" dated October 14, 1944. He envisioned a column, filled, for example, with silica and attached through its lower inlet to a flask containing a mixture of two solvents, such as methanol and toluene. This mixture is brought to a boil so that, after condensation, the vapors will establish a gradient with the highest methanol concentration at the top of the column. When a sample is introduced at the top, its components will migrate downwards until they find their respective stationary equilibrium position. In Tiselius' own words, "The advantage of the method other than the fact that 'gradient chromatography' should give very sharp bands ought to lie in the fact that very substantial amounts of liquid are circulating during the elution without necessarily causing undue zone spreading or demanding large quantities of adsorbent or solvent—the analogy with an extraction vessel is striking." I have not been able to find any evidence which indicates that Tiselius actually tried to utilize this principle in practice. In all likelihood, he foresaw many problems in constructing a capillary system that would give an optimally performing material transport. At any rate, the description offers a glance at Tiselius' way of approaching research problems—an example with great weaknesses but with a touch of genius. Many such examples are to be found in his laboratory notebooks, examples which are often naive, sometimes clever, and sometimes even marked by genius—the notes of "adult," "an ordinary researcher," or "a genius," all depending upon his state of mind. These notes express hope and curiosity, but seldom or never disappointment.

Tiselius must have followed with satisfaction how Claesson, through his gas analysis on charcoal, foreshadowed gas chromatography. Cast in a different mold, protein chromatography became successful through the pioneering work of Sober and Peterson, who introduced cellulose-based ion exchangers as adsorbents that could be eluted by means of a gradient technique along the lines developed by Tiselius and co-workers. Tiselius himself contributed, toward the end of his scientific career, to the field of protein chromatography, when, partly in collaboration with Hjertén and Levin, he studied the adsorption properties of calcium phosphate (Tiselius, 1954; Tiselius, Hjertén, and Levin, 1956).

During the 1940's, Tiselius did not completely forget his interest in electrophoresis, although other methods such as foam extraction and counter-current distribution more often occupied his mind. In 1950, he published, together with Haglund and Kunkel, some methodological descriptions of paper and column electrophoresis (Tiselius and Haglund, 1950; Tiselius and Kunkel, 1951). These led to an intense development of "zone electrophoresis"—a phrase coined by Tiselius (1953). Of particular importance are the attempts of Synge and Tiselius (1950) to take advantage of the friction caused by collodium gel. They predict that whenever transport of proteins is caused by electroosmotic flow through a dense gel, the protein molecules should be retarded with respect to the flow of the liquid due to their relative friction. The experimental results hardly measured up to expectation, but foreshadowed the very efficient gel electrophoresis methods later to be developed principally by Smithies, Ornstein, and Davies.

Many have expressed the belief that these experiments also formed the background for later work on gel chromatography. This is, however, not the case. Molecular sieving was discovered by myself in Uppsala, as I will describe below, roughly at the same time that Deuel did his work on cross-linked locust bean gum.

After receiving the Nobel Prize in 1948, Tiselius became more and more interested in problems above the molecular level, notably in virus particles and cell fragments. In his writings, he does not contribute much to this field, but he encourages other researchers to direct their attention to problems of this nature. On the local level, his interest resulted in the establishment of Sweden's first chair in molecular biology and later also a professorship in microbiology. Tiselius' great interest in Albertsson's work on polymeric phase systems should be viewed in this light. Among important contributions to the applied field I would like to mention Weibull's isolation and characterization of bacterial flagellae and ghosts. Frick's work on nucleic acids was unfortunately interrupted by his tragic and premature death.

Tiselius' contributions to biochemistry were almost exclusively confined to the methodology of separation. While being well aware of the importance of methods for the progress of science, he was sensitive to the opinion, held by many, that such research directions were limited and sterile. He always tried to excuse his special interest, and as time passed, he became successively more inclined toward declaring a strong bond between methods and applications. In his remaining notes (unpublished), one finds daring speculations about "long-range forces" and explanations of enzymatic catalysis based on the transport of energy through resonance vibrations between enzyme and substrate molecule. I am not in a position to assess the value of these speculations, but I think that his reluctance to publish these ideas constitutes an example of his common sense and the awareness of his own limitations. Like many other aspects of his work, they do, however, indicate an unusual breadth of interest and a profound interest in general scientific problems.

In his youth, he collected zeolite material at the Faroe Islands, while he later collected plants from which he extracted colored substances to use as models in his chromatographic investigations. In all likelihood, he derived as much pleasure out of observations made in a natural setting as in the laboratory.

Tiselius held a professorial chair practically free from teaching obligations. He had the unique opportunity of personally formulating the main rules for the research program: "to search for the physical laws manifested by living nature"—a wide-reaching goal that transcends the boundaries of biochemistry. I did not have the honor of hearing him lecture during my time as a student in Uppsala; it was not until 1951, during my stay in Berkeley, which coincided with an invitation to Tiselius for a guest professorship, that I had this pleasure. To many at his home institute, he became during his later years something of a "transcendent," but to me he became an increasingly close friend who opened his heart, slowly in the beginning but then more and more confidentially—a lonely man who had lost youth's naive belief in the capacity of science to relieve mankind of its plagues. For many like myself, Tiselius was, in spite of all, a great teacher of scientific methodology and theory, who was able to instill an appreciation for the technique of formulating concrete problems conducive to the progress of one's discipline. Through his personal example, he was also a teacher in scientific morality, be it endurance, an awesome respect for nature, or tolerance toward colleagues holding opinions at variance with his own. However, when he considered right or truth to be endangered, he never hesitated to face his responsibility and "sing out like the prophets of Israel." This did, on rare occasions, bring him into trouble with a number of leading Swedish scientists. Such was the case when, as a member of investigation committees, he voiced his opinion that medicobiologic fields be given priority over physics, and when he took a stand in favor of the modern molecular biology, rather than the traditional descriptive discipline, which historically has such a firm footing in Sweden. On this last issue I could not completely agree with my friend and teacher, even though I respected his opinions.

If one might detect a continuous decline in Tiselius' scientific activity, one will simultaneously register an increase in his interest and engagement in the political aspects of science, in particular those concerned with the transfer of scientific results into a form that would be of use for society. Aided by his prestige, he strongly advised Pharmacia, then only a very small pharmaceutical company, to build its future on the Ingelman-Grönwall idea of utilizing dextran as a substitute for blood plasma. Through his position as member of the Academy of Engineering Sciences and through his industrial connections, Tiselius worked for a bridging of the gap between the men of industry and of the Academy. After leaving the future of his institute in my hands, he formed, together with myself, an organization, with the two of us as shareholders, which was designed to work for transfer of research results from the Institute to industry. This nonprofit organization, which is still in existence today, combines both idealistic and practical ventures. At least 50% of the income in royalties return as research support and thereby, among other things, cover the costs for increased collaboration with foreign institutes. In our attempts to meet this goal, we have had great assistance from Professor Otto Stelling in his capacity as our "chief manager" for a number of years. The appreciation which Tiselius enjoyed in industrial circles resulted in a recognition from Alfa Laval for his achievements in the field of separation science.

Shortly after the war, Tiselius rendered his country great services through his participation in the creation of the Swedish Natural Science Research Council, whose first chairman he became. Of still greater importance became his activity within the Nobel foundation, of which he was president for a number of years. His contacts, which reached widely beyond the borders of this country, were further increased by his engagement in the Nobel foundation and the Academy of Sciences. Of particular importance was his participation in the International Union for Pure and Applied Chemistry, IUPAC, where he was first president for the biologic section, IUB, in 1947–1951; later, during a 4-year period, he acted as president of the entire union. We did not see much of Tiselius in Uppsala during this period, much to our sorrow. We missed him considerably during these years, which were also the first years of his new independent institute. His obligations toward the international community of chemists were greater than toward us. This we understood, and we regarded it as a sign of confidence that he left us so much freedom to pursue our own interests. In retrospect, one may wonder at the remarkable fact that most of us who were graduate students at that time later became professors or leaders within the Swedish chemical industry. Tiselius belonged to the category of academic teachers who believe that personal initiative is more important for scientific schooling than learning by rote under supervision.

During his later years, Tiselius became increasingly concerned over society's lack of maturity in assimilating and digesting the fruits of the tree of knowledge. He penetrated the great questions of the time and met with politicians behind all curtains. Through his straightforward and thoughtful advice he became universally appreciated and was the recipient of honorary doctorates and memberships in academies and societies all over the world. He valued and enjoyed the position as honorary president of the Electrophoretical Society of Japan as much as his membership in the papal academy, but he became increasingly aware of the responsibility which accompanied all this prestige. Tiselius was always prepared to suggest and to assist in the arrangements of symposia, conferences, and meetings in physical chemistry, biochemistry, and molecular microbiology. As a result of his initiative, the Nobel Foundation started its activities as sponsor of specialist conferences. These conferences were made financially possible through funds that became available when the

Swedish government assumed the fiscal responsibility for the future activities at the Nobel Institutes of Physics and Chemistry. According to his opinion, his most valuable contribution as a scientific politician was the initiative which led to the Nobel Foundation's conference on "The Place of Valuc in a World of Facts," which was held in Stockholm in September 1969. Tiselius preferred to stay in the background during the actual conference, but there is no doubt that he, together with his secretary, Dr. Sam Nilsson, can be largely credited for its far reaching scope. Not only natural scientists were invited, but also sociologists, futurologists, economists, authors, and politicians from all around the world.

Invited representatives of the Swedish youth served as provoking participants. He was well aware of the limited impact that one solitary conference can have in directing development toward a more human society, and, thus, he desired a continual reinforcement of the first conference's recommendations. This will be done as new Nobel conferences are arranged along similar lines.

Tiselius shared an impressive interest in everything he met in life. He could be equally as fascinated by an ordinary person as by one of the world's more important dignitaries, by every day problems as by the great events of the time, by an insignificant flower at his beloved country home as by momentous laboratory discoveries. In this universal cultural interest lies perhaps the secret of his great prestige in all quarters. His greatest nonscientific contributions were also made as a mediator in conflicts either within his own faculty, research councils, the Nobel Foundation, or on the directional boards of private foundations, banks, corporations, or international organizations. It has been witnessed by representatives of all categories, and he was well aware of his talent in this respect. A collaboration for more than 20 years without any conflict, and the deep mutual respect which existed between Tiselius and myself, form the background to the sometimes personal opinions brought forth in this article. As I see it, he underwent a personal development characterized in his youth by a desire to become a servant to science; at the height of his career, he showed a strong desire to earn a reputation as a competent scientist; and, as he reached maturity, he became increasingly aware of his responsibilities toward society, with a wish to be considered as a servant to mankind.

After this survey of Tiselius' later achievements in fields removed from actual separation science, I would like to return to a description of the activities within this field that took place at the Institute of Biochemistry after its move into new localities of its own in 1952.

After the fundamental work in electrophoresis and chromatography that had been done by Tiselius and his collaborators in the period 1930–1950, we, his pupils, continued to explore this field without any direct contact with our teacher, but with his invaluable encouragement and administrative support. The 1950's were hardly an interval of stagnation. Judged by today's experience, the discovery of gels with molecular sieving properties must be considered as the most important method which was developed by us during those years. Closely associated with these are the extraction methods based on aqueous polymer phase systems, which rank only slightly behind the former.

I have often been asked about how we discovered Sephadex. My own recollection is the following: Toward the end of the 1940's and in the early 1950's, Tiselius, Kunkel, Haglund, Flodin, and Kupke had attempted to improve the existing methods for preparative electrophoresis by performing the separation in a column filled with insoluble substances for the purpose of lowering and if possible eliminating convective material transport. I had gained some experience with electrophoresis in horizontal separation chambers filled with starch gel, which I had used during my stay as a visiting scientist in the laboratories of Professor C. H. Li in Berkeley. Together with Per Flodin, I worked out a technique for column electrophoresis using starch as the carrier medium (Flodin and Porath, 1954). The method was tested by Professor and Mrs. Siliprandi, who spent some months as visiting scientists at our Institute. In some experiments with thiamine and pyridoxal phosphates, a rather remarkable observation was made. The resolution of the cofactor components was considerably poorer than usual. Mrs. Siliprandi suspected that her husband, in his not unusual absentmindedness, had forgotten to turn on the current the night before. In the morning, he had in the usual manner performed elution of the starch column. I found these results rather perplexing. The separation was obviously the result of some chromatographic effect. Since the starch carried the same type of electric charges as the thiamine phosphates, there were two possible reasons for the separation: ionic or molecular exclusion. The latter would depend on relations between the respective molecular dimensions and the permeability of the starch. During a 3-week period, I studied the phenomenon using a wide variety of model compounds. It became evident that salts, low molecular weight sugars, and amino acids migrated with about half the velocity of albumin and other proteins. Bacitracin and a few other polypeptides that occupied my interest at the time migrated at an intermediate rate. Furthermore, I found that many dyes, although not all, migrated as discrete bands without tailing. It became obvious to me that the separation was predominantly governed by molecular size. The gel beds did, however, display some less desirable properties which I interpreted as due to bacterial growth: the effluent contained large amounts of carbohydrate and did, in time, turn strongly opaque, while the flow rate was drastically reduced. I gave up further experiments after having performed a few tests in buffers containing bacteriostatic compounds (particularly chloroform). Per Flodin told Dr. Börje Lindqvist at the Central Milk Distributing Agency in Stockholm about these experiments, and together with Torsten Storgårds Lindqvist published an article in *Nature* on peptide separations in columns packed with starch gel. The method was a year or so later, in England, employed by Lathe and Ruthven, who suggested its use for determination of molecular size. They considered the molecular sieving to reflect the special molecular structure of the starch grains.

At a somewhat later time–1956 or 1957–when Per Flodin had joined the staff at the pharmaceutical company, Pharmacia, we were discussing the anticonvection problem in preparative electrophoresis. Flodin happened to mention a dextran preparation which was made a number of years ago by Björn Ingelman. It would be both charge free and insoluble and might be of use in this context. Some days later I tried out the preparation, which in a swelled form is packed into a column, and found that dyes were migrating in discrete zones and that a mixture of phycocyan and DNP–glycine was resolved in the same manner as by the starch gel columns a number of years earlier (Porath and Flodin, 1959). The compound *Se*paration-*Pha*rmacia-*Dex*tran had been discovered. Dextran gels with different types of cross-linking were being prepared and tested. Furthermore, gels based on cellulose, polyvinylalcohol, or other hydroxyl-containing polymers were synthesized. These dextran gels proved themselves mechanically superior and were, thus, prepared for molecular sieving in different size ranges. In due time, Per Flodin presented his inaugural dissertation, which was a systematic investigation of Sephadex and gels of similar nature.

Tiselius thought the separation was caused by the relative rates of diffusion into the gel phase, exhibited by the different compounds. Already the early starch experiments had convinced me that the separation was governed by the relative accessibility of the gel phase, since I saw no other explanation for the fact that the relative migration rates were independent of the flow of the carrier ligand. My basic views on the mechanism were described in a note to one of the earliest publications (Porath, 1960). Flodin shared my mechanistic opinion and attempted to clarify his views in his dissertation. In a paper, which by now may be only of historic interest (Porath, 1963), and also at a lecture in Florence, I described how a very simple spatial model could explain the separation based on molecular size. In retrospect, it is interesting to recall the skeptical reception of this method at the institute, as well as elsewhere. One objection often raised pertained to the narrow interval of separation: could a method offering a separation range between R_f 0.5 and 1.0 really be of any practical use? I was often dismayed by the lack of understanding for the great potential lying in the use of those tailormade gels, which allowed a variation of the conditions for association or dissociation of the substances whose separation and purification is desired.

Tiselius became convinced of the advantages of the method and urged the managing director of Pharmacia, Elis Göth, to produce and market the new gel product. From this period—around 1957—dates a very fruitful collaboration between the Institute of Biochemistry and Pharmacia, which thereby extended its activities outside the pharmaceutical area.

Without the support and the interest which Stanford Moore and Lyman Craig showed in the new molecular sieving technique, it would certainly have taken considerably longer time for the method to come into focus. We have always had an open and informative relation with The Rockefeller University, a fact which has been most stimulating and gratifying. A visit by a representative from Water's Associates, who tried to introduce an interferometric method for concentration determinations in effluents from gel columns, is likely to have stimulated American scientists to develop gels for "permeation chromatography."

The second methodological area that was explored in Uppsala during this period deals with fractionation of molecules and particles in aqueous polymer phase systems and lies in the province of Per-Åke Albertsson's research activities. He became aware of this potential method for fractionation purely by accident. When he attempted to solubilize the material in chloroplasts, he found that after extraction with polyethylene glycol, the chlorophyll-containing particles concentrated in an upper-phase layer. Based on this experiment, some data on polymer two-phase systems from the literature and a theory for particle distribution between two mutually insoluble phases, which had been developed by Brønsted 30 years earlier, he set to work to develop his new method of fractionation. A meticulous study was performed on three component systems consisting of water and water-soluble polymers, such as polyethylene glycol (PEG) of different molecular weights, cellulose derivatives, and dextran with or without salts. In his inaugural dissertation, Albertsson (1960) described an impressive number of phase diagrams, which formed the background for his later developmental work. Parameters responsible for the separation are the molecular size in conjunction with the surface properties of the particles or molecules. No doubt, hydrophilic–hydrophobic interactions play a pronounced role, which has so far been only partially clarified. Particular preference for one phase or the other—or for the interphase—has been treated theoretically with strong experimental support. The Albertsson phase systems are particularly well suited for fractionation of fragile, biologically sensitive structures, such as subcellular particles and virus. They are well suited for multiple extraction, and, thus, for fractionation of particles with slight differences in surface properties, e.g., different strains of one and the same type of bacterium or erythrocytes of different age, etc. Lately, Albertsson has constructed multiphase systems, where four or more phases are in simultaneous equilibrium. In this manner, a system with graded hydrophobicity could be obtained which would enable group separations of proteins and particles. The slow breakthrough experienced by the Albertsson partitioning technique may only be explained by the development of alternative methods and by the fact that elimination of the polymers, in some cases, has constituted a problem. It is, however, the present author's conviction that the future will see an increased use of the Albertsson partitioning technique, with possible modifications to increase selectivity. Bioaffinity extraction would be one modification with considerable appeal. An enzyme inhibitor could, for instance, be attached to one of the polymers, thus enabling it to selectively complex with a soluble or particle-bound enzyme and, thereby, favor its partitioning into another phase separate from the bulk of material in a given extract.

Albertsson left Uppsala for a newly created chair in biochemistry at Sweden's northernmost university, situated in Umeå, from which he recently moved to be installed as professor at the University of Lund in southern Sweden. In Uppsala, during the 1960's, research on separation techniques continued both on electrophoresis and on gel chromatography. I received a personal chair as a research professor. When Tiselius retired, I was awarded his endowed chair, and a new professorship was created, with Stellan Hjertén as first occupant.

Hjertén was introduced to separation research in connection with Tiselius' attempts to perform protein chromatography on calcium phosphate (Tiselius *et al.*, 1956). In collaboration with Östen Levin, they found brushite to be a form of hydroxyapatite particularly well suited for this purpose. Unfortunately, linear adsorption conditions are rarely at hand, but, through a change in the eluant's phosphate concentration, one can achieve an efficient release of adsorbed proteins. One advantage of chromatography on hydroxyapatite over ion exchange resins, whether based on cellulose, Sephadex, or other polymers, is its retention of a high adsorption capacity, even in buffers of elevated ionic strength. Chromatography on hydroxyapatite, thus, constitutes a valuable tool for group separation of proteins from high-concentration salt solutions.

Concurrent with these studies was some synthesis activity on my part, which led to the production of a number of ion exchangers based on cellulose-, sulfoethyl-, sulfomethyl- and triethylaminoethylcellulose, among others (Porath, 1957a,b). Protein chromatography on these cellulose derivatives was performed, following guidelines laid down by the important work of Herbert Sober and Elbert Peterson on DEAE and CM cellulose.

Hjertén later contributed some very useful methodological work. He developed an electrophoretic method in which the separation is carried out without the use of a solid support material (Hjertén, 1958, 1967a). Gravitational convection was eliminated by a rotation of the separation chamber at a suitable speed. The principle had once been suggested by Alexander Kolin at the University of California in Los Angeles, but was never tested in practice until Hjertén gave it his attention. The Hjertén method, which is well suited for careful mobility determinations of solutes differing in character from ions to visible particles, lends itself to zone electrophoretic fractionation on a preparative scale. Solute in a microgram–milligram range can easily be handled. One of the great advantages of the Hjertén machine is the possibility to scan the sample chamber, which consists of precision bored quartz, with visible or ultraviolet light and, thus, follow the separation during the course of the experiment. With the aid of capillary plastic tubing, one can eliminate a sample (e.g., a protein-containing zone) while in the middle of a run.

Hjertén also took an interest in electrophoresis in gel stabilized media. After some early work with Sephadex, he went over to polyacrylamide (Hjertén, 1961; Hjertén and Mosbach, 1962) and agarose. In this manner, he came in contact with molecular sieving and contributed to the development of new separation media.

Hjertén soon realized one important weakness of the agarose gels: their high concentration of charged groups, which causes an extraneous electroosmosis leading to considerable losses through adsorption. By separating out the high sulfate content fraction (agaropectin), he obtained a product characterized by a very low content of matrix-bound ionic groups, which had been named agarose by Araki. Hjertén performed electrophoresis in agarose at a variety of concentrations and was able to show that excellent stabilizing effects can be obtained even with very dilute agarose suspensions. After a completed run, such suspensions can be removed from the sample chamber with a "plug flow" and collected in fractions where the polymer is eliminated from the protein solution through centrifugation.

The agarose turned out to be an excellent complement to the Sephadex gels due to their higher permeability. Hjertén showed that high molecular weight compounds, such as phycoerythrin and phycocyan, could be resolved by molecular sieving. Even subcellular particles could penetrate the gel (Hjertén, 1967b), provided the agarose content was kept sufficiently low.

During the period 1958–1962, I studied the adsorption properties of the Sephadex gels. Simultaneously with the discovery of the molecular sieving effects, we had also observed certain adsorption phenomena which were superimposed on the first effect. Bertil Gelotte of Pharmacia, also one of Tiselius' former pupils, and I both published around the same time our results from investigations on aromatic adsorption and how this effect could be reinforced or weakened (Porath, 1960; Gelotte, 1960). More in-depth studies were later carried out by David Eaker (Eaker and Porath, 1967), Nermin Fornstedt, and myself (Porath, 1968, 1969). Together with Fornstedt I discovered a phenomenon which, remarkably enough, has remained undescribed by others, namely the "halogen affinity" for strongly cross-linked Sephadex gels (Sephadex G-10, G-20, LH-Sephadex, and acetylated Sephadex derivatives). Other effects of a less pronounced nature, which reflect differences in conformation or ionic hydratization, were studied by W. Marsden at the Institute for Medical Physiology here in Uppsala. All these studies led up to our later work on hydrophobic adsorption, an area which did not come under intense study until in the 1970's when two independent groups at the Institute, led by Hjertén and myself, focused attention on this effect.

The molecular sieving gels were developed from a need for inert, insoluble supports for electrophoresis, which could swell in water. Inert gels are also suitable starting materials for production of adsorbents with well-defined properties. This formed the starting point for one work in the early 1960's aimed at the development of new bioselective adsorption methods. A year or 2 after the introduction of Sephadex, we made the first attempts at preparing adsorbents for isoagglutinins through a coupling of blood group substances to a gel with aromatic substituents containing isothiocyanate groups. These studies, which were carried out by Lennart Rhodén, Johan Killander, Per Flodin, and myself, were never published, although the coupling method was later elaborated by Axén and me for use in enzyme immobilization. It was also used to modify the Wide radioimmunoadsorption assay (Wide and Porath, 1966). During a number of years, we experimented with the avidin–biotin system to refine the technique of biospecific adsorption and desorption (Porath, 1967). We were only moderately successful, but acquired a great deal of insight into the inherent weaknesses of the experimental foundation for what has later been called "affinity chromatography." There was an obvious need for a carrier matrix with properties superior to those offered by Sephadex and cellulose, as well as for a better way to anchor the "ligand" in the matrix. An excellent coupling method was discovered through the interplay of international cooperation and a fortuitous coincidence. Rolf Axén, then recently returned from a year's visit as visiting scientist at the laboratory of Bernhard Witkop in Bethesda, suggested to one of our graduate students, Sverker Ernback, the possibility of preparing cyanamide–Sephadex through treatment of an amino derivative of Sephadex with cyanogen bromide. Cyanamide–Sephadex would then be sufficiently reactive to form guanidino bridges between an amino group containing solute and the gel. Enzymes turned out to be easily immobilized in high yields and with good retention of activity. When Ernback showed me the results of some model couplings of dipeptides, I noticed that considerably more peptide was attached than one would have anticipated from the original gel content of the amino groups. Control experiments involving unsubstituted Sephadex confirmed the suspicion that cyanogen bromide reacted with the polysaccharide matrix, leading to the formation of a reactive derivative which coupled amino acids, peptides, and proteins (Axén *et al.*, 1967). The reaction has later been studied in detail by Axén and coworkers.

At about the same time, we set off on a search for suitable gel matrices. Cellulose in different forms was tested (mercerized, acid treated, precipitated from xanthates, etc.), as were cross-linked polyvinylalcohol, polyacrylamide, and Sephadex, but none was found to be satisfactory. Finally, we settled for agarose (Porath *et al.*, 1967), to which enzymes were immobilized with the cyanogen bromide coupling method.

Around this time, a debate had started at the Institute concerning its contemplated future course of action. Three directions of interest had crystallized, one led by the remaining students of Professor Hans Boman who had moved north to Umeå, and the other two spearheaded by Hjertén and myself. The first of these groups favored a strong emphasis on molecular biology, while it was my opinion that we should concentrate on methods for biospecific adsorption, protein characterization, and peptide synthesis. My strongest supporters in these discussions were Karin Caldwell and Arne Tiselius. Hjertén preferred to focus his research efforts on the fractionation and characterization of membranous fragments.

Together with Tore Kristiansen and Lars Sundberg, I showed that we were now in an excellent position for the preparation of biospecific adsorbents (Porath, 1968). The cyanogen bromide method could be used, not only for coupling of amino derivatives, but also hydroxyl group containing substances as well, such as carbohydrates, provided a diamine was used as an intermediary (Kristiansen *et al.*, 1969). We managed to successfully carry out a number of chromatographic experiments involving, on one hand, isoagglutinins and blood group substance A, and, on the other, enzymes and enzyme inhibitors, particularly soya bean inhibitor in conjunction with pancreatic extracts. As it turned out, we were superseded in our efforts by Pedro Cuatrecasas, Meir Wilchek, and Chris Anfinsen in

Bethesda. They had adopted our methods, and, in a brilliant study, were able to demonstrate their usefulness for an efficient selective fractionation of enzymes through the use of low molecular weight substrate analogues of a peptide nature, or of inhibitors attached to agarose through the cyanogen bromide method. During the years that followed up to the present, we have spent much time and effort on attempts to improve the agarose matrix (Porath *et al.,* 1971, 1975a) and to introduce new and complementary coupling methods (Porath and Sundberg, 1970; Axén *et al.,* 1971; Sundberg and Porath, 1974; Porath and Axén, 1977). In some cases, these have proved to be superior. Model studies on immunosorptive methods for the isolation of antibodies and antigens have been carried out in collaboration with Hormone Research Laboratory in San Francisco and Institut de Recherches Cliniques de Montréal. Model studies of bioadsorption with the use of lectin gels also constitute part of the work to develop new selective methods for the development of glycoproteins (Aspberg and Porath, 1970; Ersson *et al.,* 1973; Ersson and Porath, 1974).

Throughly impressed by the enormous simplification in the separation procedure, which is often provided by the affinity chromatography, a great number of people have allowed their interest in new general methods of fractionation to dwindle. We do, however, still consider it highly desirable to work both for an improvement in already existing conventional methods and for the introduction of other methods based on new parameters. It is in this vein that the author has devoted much interest on side chain selective methods for fractionation of protein and peptides. A recent example along these lines is given by the metal chelate gels, which near neutral pH display a particularly strong affinity toward histidyl side chains (Porath *et al.,* 1975b). Among other less selective procedures, one might mention hydrophobic adsorption chromatography (Porath *et al.,* 1973; Hjertén, 1973; Rosengren *et al.,* 1975) and methods based on charge-transfer adsorption—the latter so far having met with modest success (Porath and Caldwell, 1976, 1977). These areas are currently studied by Dr. Karin Caldwell, a pupil of mine and of J. C. Giddings at the University of Utah in Salt Lake City, in a joint project. Finally, I would like to mention "covalent chromatography," an area with which we have had increasing contact as the result of a collaboration between Dr. Brocklehurst in Professor Eric Crook's group in London and Jan Carlsson and Rolf Axén of my laboratory (Carlsson *et al.,* 1976). So far, methods based on thiol–disulfide exchange have been the most successful.

I have tried to account for the most successful of the publicized discoveries and innovations in the field of separation science which have originated from the Uppsala Institute of Biochemistry and which have enjoyed a universal recognition. At the Institute, there has accumulated over the years a substantial amount of knowledge, which so far has not been published, or which has evoked only limited attention, but which is often helpful in providing guidelines for scientific planning here. A strong reservation against publication is an old tradition for better or for worse. In retrospect, it is interesting to analyze its consequences; as an example, I would like to quote the following from the laboratory journal of Arne Tiselius, dated September 20, 1929: "Preliminary experiments concerning a biochemically and medically suited cathaphoresis method, aiming at the investigation of biological fluids with respect to different proteins, antibodies and possibly enzymes ('electrophoretic analysis').

Cataphoresis in gels offers the possibility of working at higher voltages and with substances in concentrations as low as those of antibodies and enzymes, without disturbing heat convection. Furthermore, this opens the possibility for the development of a completely new kind of technique, based on the following principle:

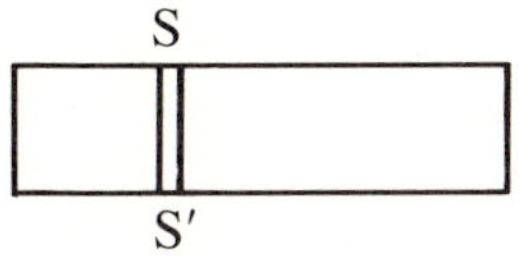

A glass plate is coated with a thin layer of gel, e.g., agar, containing a suitable buffer. Within the gel is made a narrow slot, SS′, which is filled with a protein mixture in the same buffer (one can also make a scratch with a pen dipped in the solution, 11–10–29). The plate is then connected with electrode vessels, and a suitably high voltage is applied. As a result of the migration of the proteins and the endoosmosis through the gel, these proteins will be transported through the gel in the shape of lines which are split into separate bands as a result of differences in the rates of migration. These might be identified in different ways . . ."

On September 21, 1929, Tiselius made one experiment using a 1% gelatin solution and a mixture of phycocyan and phycoerythrin in phosphate solution in his "old electrophoresis machine." He achieved the desired separation of the colored proteins and noted in his book: "Fundamental experiment, demonstrated correctness of the assumption which forms the basis for the proposed technique." Somewhat later, Tiselius described how he had succeeded in separating different protein mixtures in gelatin and agar, and in fixing and staining them. He interrupted his experiments but resumed them again 2 years later, in October 1931. At this time he worked with much higher gelatin concentrations. Soon, however, he switched over to use Willstätter's aluminum oxide gels. It is interesting to note that at this time he used a fluorometer to localize the protein zones. He also carried out electrophoresis of phycoerythrin adsorbed to an Al_2O_3 gel, and, thus, finished this series of experiments, which were never published.

Personally, I have rarely encountered unpublished work of such fundamental importance. Pioneering experiments with volatile buffer systems (Porath, 1955), zonal precipitation (Porath, 1962), ion exclusion (Porath and Lindner, 1961), continuous concentration, and dialysis of the effluent from a chromatographic column have all been described in short communications, and have been incorporated into commonly practiced biochemical techniques. I am pleased to note that step-graded columns (Porath, 1954), which were once suggested by me for group separations involving active charcoal, are now in existence in a version designed by Shaltiel, who uses hydrophobic chromatography for the separation of proteins.

Molecular sieving chromatography has an inherent weakness in the narrowness of its separation interval. The ratio of the difference between the elution and void volumes and the total volume of the gel bed, $V_e - V_o/V_T$, varies between zero and an upper limit less than one. This limitation can to a large degree be compensated by using a series of gel beds with decreasing molecular exclusion limits. Another possible way to improve resolution is to increase the height of the gel bed (leading to a larger number of theoretical plates). A limit to the bed height was set by the compressibility of the gels, leading to a compacting of the beds and resulting low flow rates. Another effect counteracting the separation arises from inhomogeneity throughout the gel bed. Bennich and I suggested a connection between the extremeties of a column and a recycling of the material in the zones through pumping of the eluant (Porath and Bennich, 1962). Zonal migration would be controlled through a monitoring of the UV absorbance of the effluent in the external free liquid. Nermin Fornstedt and I made a very thorough investigation of the packing conditions in beds of different dimensions, using gel particles of different diameters and size distributions. We also investigated the zone broadening and its dependence on the rate of flow. The work took on substantial proportions and the experimental material eventually became so unwieldy that no collective publication was made. Sporadically, we have had occasion to make reference to these systematic investigations. We found, for instance, that the plate heights were minimal for bed heights ranging from 15 to 30 cm and for column diameters in the range 5–7 cm. Based on these results, Jan-Christer Janson and I attached a series of gel beds to each other in the form of stack columns of considerable size (5 × 30 liters). Pharmacia adopted the idea, and columns of this type are currently available commercially.

At the Seventh International Symposium on Gas Chromatography in

Copenhagen 1968, (Porath, 1969) I gave an account for some adsorption and sieving properties of LH-Sephadex. By using three consecutive columns of LH-Sephadex in 96% ethanol, a mixture of oligomers of monophenyl ethylene glycols were completely resolved up to the dodecamer, a result which anticipates the forthcoming of high efficiency liquid chromatography.

Electrophoresis in mixed solvents was performed by Störiko and myself (Porath and Störiko, 1962), using simple model substances. The method has so far not been particularly well developed, but should, in one form or other, be of use in the fractionation of membrane proteins. Dextran-bounded insulin and antibiotic peptides, as well as cross-linked artificial enzyme complexes were prepared in collaboration with Rolf Axén and Per Vretblad, but the results were never published, even though the work also lies on the side of the actual separation research.

Those pupils of Tiselius who left the Institute have also made important contributions, before and after. In particular, I want to mention Harry Svensson-Rilbe. As Tiselius' student, he developed and refined moving boundary electrophoresis (Svensson, 1946). He introduced continuous preparative electrophoresis (Svensson and Brattsten, 1949), together with Inger Brattsten—a technique which has also been developed to perfection by Kurt Hannig in Munich. After leaving Uppsala, Rilbe continued to develop techniques for protein separations by electric fields; his most well known contributions are density gradient electrophoresis and isoelectric focusing. Through this work, he followed in the footsteps of Tiselius.

Now that Tiselius' institute has ceased to exist, or, rather, has been transformed into one part of a larger institute at the Biomedical Center in Uppsala, the question of our future research direction has come to be of paramount importance. To the extent that University and Governmental administration will permit, we are prepared to maintain and enlarge the tradition founded by Svedberg and Tiselius. The discipline is such that its possibilities do not seem exhaustible within the foreseeable future. Among its unquestionable advantages we count the fact that we, the promulgators of that tradition, enjoy constant stimulation through our international contacts with colleagues all over the world, and through the mutual exchange of ideas resulting therefrom. This compensates for what many observers might consider a lack of continuity in the form of well-defined, limited research projects.

Tiselius, like Hjertén and myself, was always quite anxious that the methods of separations be used here at the institute to some problems of current interest. Two contacts have been of particular importance for the institute's applied research: (a) Tiselius' contacts with E. Kabat and M. Heidelberger in the 1930's, which highly stimulated the interest in

γ-globulins and immunochemistry, and (b) Tiselius' and my own contact with Professor C. H. Li in the late 1940's and early 1950's which formed the background for our work on the chemistry of the pituitary hormones. The greatest contributions in these areas were no doubt made in the laboratories of the respective researchers, with the use of our methods, rather than in Uppsala. The isolation of immunoglobulin E by Hans Bennich and G. Johansson does, however, constitute one of the most important results of our research throughout the years. In later times, I have resumed and intensified collaboration with Li and his co-workers at the Hormone Research Laboratory, and in particular with T. Bewley and M. R. Sairam, who is now in Montréal. Our aim has been the development of better immunosorptive methods for isolation of the pituitary hormones and their antibodies. I consider this collaboration as a model for international cooperation in accordance with the best traditions at the Institute of Biochemistry in Uppsala.

References

Albertsson, P. Å. (1960). "Partition of Cell Particles and Macromolecules." Almqvist & Wiksell, Stockholm.

Alm, R. S., Williams, R. J. P., and Tiselius, A. (1952). *Acta Chem. Scand.* **6,** 826–838.

Aspberg, K., and Porath, J. (1970). *Acta Chem. Scand.* **24,** 1839.

Axén, R., Porath, J., and Ernback, S. (1967). *Nature (London)* **214,** 1302.

Axén, R., Vretblad, P., and Porath, J. (1971). *Acta Chem. Scand.* **25,** 1129.

Carlsson, J., Olsson, I., Axén, R., and Drevin, H. (1976). *Acta Chem. Scand., Ser. B* **30,** 180.

Eaker, D., and Porath, J. (1967). *Separ. Sci.* **2,** 507–550.

Ersson, B., and Porath, J. (1974). *FEBS Lett.* **48,** 126.

Ersson, B., Aspberg, K., and Porath, J. (1973). *Biochim. Biophys. Acta* **310,** 446.

Flodin, P., and Porath, J. (1954). *Biochim. Biophys. Acta* **13,** 175.

Gelotte, B. (1960). *J. Chromatogr.* **3,** 330.

Hjertén, S. (1958). *Ark. Kemi* **13,** 151.

Hjertén, S. (1961). *Biochim. Biophys. Acta* **53,** 514.

Hjertén, S., and Mosbach, R. (1962). *Anal. Biochem.* **3,** 109.

Hjertén, S. (1967a). *Chromatogr. Rev.* **9,** 122.

Hjertén, S. (1967b). *Protides Biol. Fluids, Proc. Colloq.* **14,** 553.

Hjertén, S. (1973). *J. Chromatogr.* **87,** 325.

Keckwick, R. A., and Pedersen, K. O. (1974). *Biogr. Mem. Fellows R. Soc.* **20,** 401–428.

Kristiansen, T., Sundberg, L., and Porath, J. (1969). *Biochim. Biophys. Acta* **184,** 93.

Porath, J. (1954). *Ark. Kemi.* **7,** No. 57.

Porath, J. (1955). *Nature (London)* **175,** 478.

Porath, J. (1957a). *Ark. Kemi* **11,** No. 11.

Porath, J. (1957b). Dissertation, Uppsala.

Porath, J. (1960). *Biochim. Biophys. Acta* **39,** 193.

Porath, J. (1962). *Nature (London)* **196,** 47.

Porath, J. (1963). *Pure Appl. Chem.* **6,** 233.

Porath, J. (1967). *Gamma Globulins, Proc. Nobel Symp., 3rd, 1967.*
Porath, J. (1968). *Nature (London)* **218,** 883.
Porath, J. (1969). *Gas Chromatogr., Proc. Int. Symp., 7th. 1968* pp. 201–216.
Porath, J., and Axén, R. (1976). *In* "Methods in Enzymology" (K. Mosbach, ed., Vol. 44, p. 19. Academic Press, New York.
Porath, J., and Bennich, H. (1962). *Arch. Biochem. Biophys., Suppl.* **1,** 152.
Porath, J., and Caldwell, K. (1976). "Conference on Biotechnical Applications of Proteins and Enzymes. On the Occasion of the 60th Birthday of Ephraim Katzir" (in press).
Porath, J., and Caldwell, K. (1977). To be published.
Porath, J., and Flodin, P. (1959). *Nature (London)* **183,** 1657.
Porath, J., and Lindner, E. B. (1961). *Nature (London)* **191,** 69.
Porath, J., and Störiko, K. (1962). *J. Chromatogr.* **7,** 385.
Porath, J., and Sundberg, L. (1970). *Protides Biol. Fluids, Proc. Colloq.,* **18,** 401.
Porath, J., Axén, R., and Ernback, S. (1967). *Nature (London)* **215,** 1491.
Porath, J., Janson, J. –C., and Låås, T. (1971). *J. Chromatogr.* **60,** 167.
Porath, J., Sundberg, L., Fornstedt, N., and Olsson, I. (1973). *Nature (London)* **245,** 465.
Porath, J., Låås, T., and Janson, J. –C. (1975a). *J. Chromatogr.* **103,** 49.
Porath, J., Carlsson, J., Olsson, I., and Belfrage, G. (1975b). *Nature (London)* **258,** 598.
Rosengren, J., Påhlman, S., Glad, M., and Hjertén, S. (1975). *Biochim. Biophys. Acta* **412,** 51.
Sundberg, L., and Porath, J. (1974). *J. Chromatogr.* **90,** 87.
Svedberg, T., and Tiselius, A. (1926). *J. Am. Chem. Soc.* **48,** 2272–2278.
Svensson, H. (1946). *Ark. Kemi, Mineral. Geol.* **22A,** No. 10.
Svensson, H., and Brattsten, I. (1949). *Ark. Kemi* **1,** 401.
Synge, R. L. M., and Tiselius, A. (1950). *Biochem. J.* **46,** xli–xlii.
Tiselius, A. (1926). *Z. Phys. Chem.* **124,** 449–463.
Tiselius, A. (1927). *In* "Handbuch der biologischen Arbeitsmethoden" (E. Abderhalden, ed., Vol. III B, pp. 629–678. Urban & Schwarzenberg, Berlin.
Tiselius, A. (1930). *Nova Acta Regiae Soc. Sci. Ups.* [4] **7,** No. 4, 1–107.
Tiselius, A. (1932). *Kolloid-Z.* **59,** 306–309.
Tiselius, A. (1936). *J. Phys. Chem.* **40,** 223–232.
Tiselius, A. (1937a). *Trans. Faraday Soc.* **33,** 524–531.
Tiselius, A. (1937b). *Biochem. J.* **31,** 313–317.
Tiselius, A. (1937c). *Biochem. J.* **31,** 1464–1477.
Tiselius, A. (1940). *Ark. Kemi, Mineral. Geol.* **14B,** No. 23, 1–5.
Tiselius, A. (1943). *Kolloid-Z.* **105,** 101–109.
Tiselius, A. (1953). *Discuss. Faraday Soc.* **13,** 29–33.
Tiselius, A. (1954). *Ark. Kemi* **7,** 443–449.
Tiselius, A. (1968). *Annu. Rev. Biochem.* **37,** 1–24.
Tiselius, A., and Hagdahl, L. (1950). *Acta Chem. Scand.* **4,** 394–395.
Tiselius, A., and Haglund, H. (1950). *Acta Chem. Scand.* **4,** 957–962.
Tiselius, A., and Horsfall, F. L., Dr. (1939). *J. Exp. Med.* **69,** 119–131.
Tiselius, A., and Kabat, E. (1938). *Science* **87,** 416–417.
Tiselius, A., and Kunkel, H. G. (1951). *J. Gen. Physiol.* **35,** 89–118.
Tiselius, A., Hjertén, S., and Levin, Ö. (1956). *Arch. Biochem. Biophys.* **65,** 132.
Wide, L., and Porath, J. (1966). *Biochim. Biophys. Acta* **130,** 257.

Author Index

Numbers in italics refer to the pages on which the complete references are listed.

M

N

O

P

T

Subject Index

V

W

Z

A 8
B 9
C 0
D 1
E 2
F 3
G 4
H 5
I 6
J 7